AWARENESS RECOVERY

Planning Your Exit Strategy for Life
After Rehab

(Last Edition)

Dael Freeman

Published By KDP Digital Publishers
www.kdpdigitalpublishers.com

KDP
WHERE STORIES COME ALIVE

ISBN
Paperback : 979-8-9905801-9-0

LCCN: 2025905829

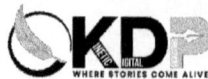

DEDICATION

Awareness Recovery is dedicated with love to my parents. They made all the blessings of my life possible. Also, to those who still suffer addiction and substance abuse.

True Life Transformations

"Three things never long hidden are the sun, the moon, and the truth."

BUDDHA

Contents

Preface

THIS I KNOW. LIFE AFTER REHAB IS AN OPPORTUNITY TO OPEN A NEW CHAPTER IN LIFE. This could mean a clean slate and a new beginning if the challenge to live sober is fully embraced. And that means growth in most areas of life.

Awareness is what needs to be recovered after living barely conscious due to substance abuse. We do not need to recover the addiction, as in the commonly used term "addiction recovery." The challenge for alcoholics and addicts is to become consciously aware of actions, beliefs, and thoughts - to be mindful of self and society.

An exit strategy is the plan you make for living a better, happier life after rehab and leaving less than desirable circumstances behind. An individual without an exit strategy could enter a dumpster fire of a life and be in a world of hurt, or at minimum, in a pitifully distressing predicament with a jigsaw puzzle of problems.

People released from professional treatment facilities for substance abuse after 30 to 90 days need support in living sober. Self-help groups like AA or SMART are helpful but do not allow a person opportunity to discuss the other stuff that life consists of, like relationships, children, money issues, and balancing life by setting priorities and objectives. That's why I work as a Life Coach for persons in recovery.

Planning an exit strategy will allow people in treatment for substance abuse, recently released from a treatment center or correctional facility, to set realistic goals and plan the steps to get there. This book will help those who once abused alcohol and drugs to live a productive, successful, and happy life sober through frequent accomplishment. Living sober is the first accomplishment.

This book was written because many people who are in rehab or incarcerated do not give careful thought to what they will do upon release. Most will daydream, and those daydreams are drawn upon memories of the past, answering questions like, "What will the house look like these days?" or "Will we still be in love?" or "I wonder what my children think of me?"

Is that you? Then you know that time in the world did not stop when you entered rehab. Everything else is changing, and now it's time for you to change, too. There is no way to live in the past. There is only now. Tomorrow never comes. It is always today. It is best to get busy preparing for your future. Plan an exit strategy that will satisfy your soul and ease potential stress after your release from rehab.

Awareness Recovery informs the reader of options to consider in the reconstruction of their life in the absence of mind-altering substances. Points of view, principles, and plans of action presented herein introduce ideas from SMART, RR, and AA.

A person seeking a drug-free future should know of as many options as there are for support that will be helpful in their sobriety.

If a member of AA is asked, "What should a person do to stay sober?" it will always be suggested that the individual go to a twelve-step meeting. If a Christian is asked what a person should do to maintain abstinence, they will be advised to go to church. Both suggestions require a faith and belief in a Higher Power or God.

Can an atheist, agnostic, or humanist stay sober? Can a Buddhist, a Jew, or a Hindu? Of course, they can! Awareness Recovery considers all addicts without regard to religious conviction or spiritual belief. No faith or lack of faith is discredited.

A Christian God is not a prerequisite for sober living. It is not reasonable to think that an atheist will obey the rules of an invisible supernatural God. Atheists are not built that way.

Meeting with other persons with addiction will be more helpful. Camaraderie is very helpful.

Not all meetings are the same, and just as every place of

worship is a different experience, so are Anonymous, SMART, and other meetings. One must visit a few to decide where is comfortable.

Aside from being able to share experiences and ideas and make small talk with like-minded people, the usually reclusive and secretive addict is now able to socialize with people who are not selling drinks or drugs. That is a positive aspect of meetings of any sober sort. Whether we choose AA, church services, SMART, or Toastmasters, it is beneficial to socialize.

The hours that were consumed each day in a state of wasted consciousness must be replaced; now, the individual becomes engaged in productive projects and daily tasks that are personally fulfilling and accomplishes desired goals. Any behavior that results in the old, unfocused, unproductive, and lazy lifestyle will cause failure in bringing happiness and, enthusiasm, and success.

Awareness Recovery suggests a practical and holistic way of life be adopted. We must become willing to accept and embrace the challenge of change. Whatever spiritual or psychological transformation is necessary to achieve total abstinence must be made.

The person seeking sobriety will struggle to gain control of their sanity. "Indeed, there is nothing more difficult to control than the mind," Dr. David Frawley writes in Ayurveda and the Mind. He adds, "Inability to control the mind causes sorrow and is behind the disease process."

Awareness Recovery motivates us by offering a myriad of ideas and stimulating suggestions to consider. Recovery from substance abuse is an arduous and, at times, seemingly insufferable battle, but it is one that can be won. Knowing that the enemy, our addictive self, is deceptive, ruthless, and does not care about lifting our consciousness up is why self-awareness is crucial. Knowing one's self is of the essence. It is the highest imperative and vitally essential to lift our consciousness to conquer, vanquish, and destroy our addiction. This victory brings glory.

The more aware and knowledgeable we are of ourselves, the better prepared we are for anything life presents. Knowledge shuns regret. When we do something that we know we should not do, it is intuitive comprehension that tells us we have done wrong. Going against our better senses and higher intuitive self always results in regret and grief. Our indiscretions never go unpunished. We always bring harmful repercussions and bad fate to our self. We sabotage our higher self due to lack of discipline and the inability to control our mind and, thus, our actions.

This is the way it is in recovery. Once we know better, doing something that is wrong anyway is dumb, really stupid. And we know it. We don't have to think about it. Intuitively, we know we did wrong. Someone got harmed. The behavior went against and was contradictory to our morality. When we engage in unethical behavior and thoughts we diminish our integrity.

This causes embarrassment, which is humiliating and disgraceful, and any witness to this foolishness will say, "Shame on you!" And we feel ashamed. The addiction has won. We want to drink or drug the shame away. We admit defeat and surrender.

We cannot win this way.

In the war against addiction, a battle is lost when we fail the higher standards of our consciousness. We have failed to use the energy of the Source with wisdom. The Source is most commonly named God as Creator amongst Christians, and Allah amongst those of Islamic faith, and other names are used by other religious faiths. The word Source is used in this book to make the explanations of our spiritual life experiences nonreligious, nondenominational, and accessible to all.

Do the right thing. Make certain every decision and action is one that is admirable. Be a role model to others.

Awareness Recovery will help you stay on the right track. War plans always need to have an exit strategy. Awareness recovery requires raising our consciousness and is our strategy to defeat addictions.

While reading this book, keep a journal of ideas. Inspiring insights will spring intuitively at times from out of the blue. That hunch or what is correct and true comes from our higher consciousness. Write that notion down. It is most likely to become an integral piece of your exit strategy. As quickly as it came it will evaporate into the unknowable ether. Therefore, you must write these thoughts down. Thoughts are like dreams. In minutes or some in a few days, they are forgotten.

Mind, Body, Spirit, and Emotional health are all vital, and all need care. Your whole person must be considered. Every type of substance abuse damages all four of these components that comprise you. By experimenting with new ideas and practicing healthy habits daily, healing will come. The objective is to become the best version of you that has ever existed.

This recovery is about healing Mind, Body, and Spirit. This strategy of expanding and uplifting your consciousness is the surest way to victory.

You will discover much about yourself in the weeks ahead. You will find your greater purpose. You will explore new beliefs. You will enthusiastically embrace challenges as you enter a new way of life. You will deepen your connection to Source.

INTRODUCTION

"If my mind can conceive it, and my heart can believe it, then I can achieve it."

- **MUHAMMAD ALI**, Heavyweight boxing champion

CONSIDER THIS BOOK A MANUAL of practical and philosophical suggestions to sustain sobriety.

Awareness Recovery discusses beliefs and principles. This is intended to challenge the reader to open their minds and hearts and expand and raise their consciousness. The terms higher-self, higher consciousness, and God-consciousness are used interchangeably, as are the terms Universe, Source, and God.

There is a lot of discussion of addiction, and, in particular, alcohol and its history in America.

In the "Addiction" chapter of The Founders on Religion: A Book of Quotations, edited by James Hutson, Hutson introduces the letters of Charles Carroll to his alcoholic son:

The younger Carroll, as his anguished father frequently reminded him, had been the beneficiary of everything that wealth and parental affection could provide: financial security, a good education, and an impressive home. In addition, Carroll, Jr., married a model wife from an excellent Philadelphia family... But the younger Carroll could not conquer his addiction to alcohol, which wrecked his life. Charles Adams, the second son of John and Abigail Adams, was also an alcoholic who died young and in disgrace.

Alcoholism has a long history of ruining lives. Few, if any, presidents of the United States have been completely sober. President Bill Clinton said he smoked marijuana, but he did not inhale. President George W. Bush had an alcohol abuse problem in his National Guard years. It became known that President Kennedy was injecting drugs for pain while in office. Franklin Roosevelt drank daily during the Prohibition years. President Barack Obama confessed to his marijuana and cocaine use in one or more of his biographies. When asked if he inhaled, Barack answered, "That's the point, isn't it?"

Presidents are only human. And not only is forgetfulness common, but memory loss is medically proven amongst substance users/abusers. So, it is possible that a president could forget to, or not even think to, ask a military general, "What's the plan for getting out? What is our exit strategy?"

The American military's sudden exits from Vietnam, Somalia, Korea, and Iraq were all hasty affairs, demonstrating poor planning and sometimes none at all. The United States never planned to lose a battle. Forgetting or neglecting to plan ahead and consider the options frequently results in unhappy consequences.

Have you had enough unhappy consequences?

Hasty and hurried, rash and brash decisions are common under the influence of mind-altering chemicals. You need to make informed and intelligent decisions when planning for the future. This is done much better sober.

Alcohol and drugs cause memory loss. Forgetting that an exit strategy is needed when going to battle could happen to any drunk or junkie. Have you ever forgotten to get a ride home or even forgotten where your car is, or, worse yet, where you are?

These scenarios never happen when sober. Without an exit strategy, you may find yourself making a last stand in a hospital or worse. That's kind of where you are now.

An indefinable mystery, a nebulous enigma, describes you and your life now. You don't know what will happen next. You worry about the future. Why? Because you do not have a clue what you will do. Hopefully, the chapters that follow will help.

Now, you are in a conundrum when it comes to life itself. What will you do? What you want to do probably is still not what you must do. The first challenge for you is to get the courage to do what has to be done. You must quit abusing alcohol and drugs.

Drug and alcohol abuse have enslaved you mentally and debilitated you physically. Your entire being is in peril. Most substance abusers prefer to remain in denial about the dark future that waits if they do not stop using.

Why not just stop? Fight for your freedom from dependency.

Global warfare is a suitable analogy for any person's internal war on drugs. The person in the battle against substance abuse must be prepared to go the distance. Victory is the objective. There is no stalemate, draw, or tie game in recovery. Stalemate only happens in chess, and very rarely. There is either abstinence or not - and so more abuse.

Do you believe life is a game? Recovery is not a game. For many reading this book, addiction and overcoming addiction is a life-or-death struggle. Continuing to play could kill you. Get real if you want to live. If you have choices, then why do you choose to live with reckless abandon? Do you think you will get a second chance, or a third? How many chances do you want?

If you do believe life is a game, you need to know that's a lazy belief. You must be a lazy person to believe this is a game. You must be soft - either soft in the head or soft in the ass, or both. Only in America can a person eat a bucket of fried chicken, watch a movie on a widescreen TV in an air-conditioned room with a smartphone on Facebook, smoke crack cocaine, drink vodka like water, and complain they are poor!

That doesn't describe you. Does it?

This book should be read when the reader is in an open state of mind.

Being emotionally vulnerable and open to new ideas, feeling anxious and challenged, is a good way to start learning. That's how most people felt on their first day of elementary school, the first day of high school, and the first day of college, on their first day in jail or in rehab. This nervousness exists as motivation, and the need to overcome fear will summon courage and generate a desire to win within you. Have you ever heard athletes comment that they feel butterflies in their stomach before a big event? That's the nervousness that motivates winners. There can be little emotional or spiritual growth when you are in your comfort zone.

The future for you is either victory or defeat. That is true. Perceive the effort you make as a constructive experience for character building. To succeed in anything that is worthwhile requires effort.

You may drink a beer one day after rehab and think, "Why am I drinking a beer? I want tequila shots! Oh well, no sense in stopping now. Just give me the bottle!"

And you may do that. That's okay. At least you thought about it and believed that it was the wrong thing for you to be doing. The next morning, you will probably know that beer and tequila was completely wrong for you! You lost that round. Forgive yourself - and hopefully, you did not binge to the extent that you return to cravings and obsession or even delirium tremens (DTs).

While in treatment for substance abuse, read Awareness Recovery in the evenings, after daytime therapy, counseling, and recreational and educational activities are done. Awareness Recovery needs to be read thoroughly and completely: front to back, with a highlighter and a notepad or journal. This is the way that things you learn during the day and the ideas in this book become unified in your own mind. Write down what strikes you as important while the insights you gain and the ideas and understanding you reach are fresh. Greater intuition will come and present sudden moments of enlightenment that will be inspiring.

Writing things down greatly helps you retain information. And you will have notes that you can refer to later. Thoughts really are like dreams, forgotten within a few minutes. Have you ever been in a conversation and had to ask, "What was I talking about?" Writing things down also keeps your mind focused. Everyone has let their mind drift in a situation and, after thirty minutes, had no idea what happened or was said.

Do you have a plan for the future? Goals will be realized with a plan. Now, with renewed ambition and self-motivation, the new you will be revealed.

Living without a plan is the way we usually lived when high all the time. Procrastination would keep most of the plans we did make from ever happening. You are finally clean and hopefully beginning to enjoy being clear of mind and physically healthy again. Hopefully you want to maintain this sober reality.

Make one plan. Plans change. That is okay. The plan need not be elaborate. The exit strategy you create needs to be simple and practical. It needs to be doable. The plan is for you. It is very personal. This is your life.

Without a plan for the future, what are you planning, then? Are you planning to return to rehab? When? Is next year too soon? Can you imagine it taking eight more years or longer to finally quit drinking and drugging: committing slow suicide? How many disasters will occur in that time? New arrests, long probation periods, long jail time - are all possible fates. You have heard the saying that failing to plan is planning to fail.

An exit strategy is what a person needs to have when leaving rehab to continue sober living in a sane and rational manner.

One way to stay free from drink and drugs is to stay active and keep learning new things. Stay curious. Develop a yearning for learning. Get motivated! Stay clean and free now. This is a great life purpose, a sane objective, and a worthwhile goal.

Aside from keeping notes about recovery and working on your plan, keep a daily journal, because writing down your thoughts are really the best way to recall or remember anything. Remember, your thoughts are like last night's dreams. They disappear quickly from the mind.

Recovery can seem boring, but sobriety is not the ultimate

goal. That's correct. Instead, sobriety is the way to become a fully functional and contributing member of society. Can you imagine that for yourself?

The notes that you write will become the fuel for developing the plans and strategies you will use to accomplish your goals. Thoughts are easily forgotten forever, lost, and they seldom return. That is why it is important to write. People in business write business plans, screenwriters write dialogue, pastors write sermons, authors write books, and songwriters write lyrics. Sending text messages does not count as writing.

When you are no longer supervised daily, as you are in rehab (or jail), you will want your own rigid, rigorous routine and rules, too. Be tough with yourself.

Write down your own rules of conduct. One rule might be "I will not forget." That way, you won't say, "I forgot!" I forgot what time it is. I forgot what day it is. I forgot to pay the electric bill. I forgot to buckle my seatbelt.

The judges and law enforcement authorities will be hard on you if you are not hard on yourself.

The details of an individualized exit strategy can be best codified and organized with the mentoring of a spiritual guide, a substance abuse counselor, a psychotherapist, a recovery life coach, or even a Twelve Step sponsor that is knowledgeable and suitable. Ask questions and ask for opinions from these people. If one of them says something that is important, write it down, either in your personal journal or in your exit strategy planner.

Successful recovery means long-term abstinence from mind-altering substances and a sober mind: freedom from alcoholism and addiction. Awareness recovery comes by building healthy new habits and life skills. You will be coping with, dealing with, and handling the truth from now on, and going forward maturely and responsibly. Rehab does not always emphasize the need for a new lifestyle behind the cessation of substance abuse and relief from chemical dependency. This is an error or an oversight. Perhaps they do not want to offend paying clients or create tension between counselors and clients by telling a client that they must change their way of living.

The truth is that being free from alcohol and drugs is only the beginning for a fresh start.

Many substance abusers do not know what to do with their life going forward. By setting goals that are realistic, you will be able to put in motion the actions needed to be successful and to complete what you want to accomplish. The exit strategy you develop will keep you on track. The goals you create will remain foremost in your mind during your daily efforts. Happiness is achieved through accomplishment. Once you are happy, then you are open to receiving all the good the Universe has for you. Like attract like, so you've got to get happy to bring joy. Step one is to get something done.

Ideas for new activities and new perspectives are offered throughout *Awareness Recovery*.

Consider new ideas and hobbies to integrate into your new lifestyle. This brings freshness and enthusiasm and will spark creative thinking, too. The whole objective is to become a functioning and contributing member of society. Someone people want to be with. Taking away the mind-altering chemicals is of no use if we remain a mean and immoral, cheating and lying thief. If you remain sober for the next ten years but make a career of bank robbery and identity theft, did the substance abuse recovery program work? Did it prevent you from a life of crime and possible incarceration? The recovery program did not work because your awareness of your own consciousness remained in the bowels of immorality.

All you accomplished was abstinence. You left intact all the flaws associated with low self-esteem. The inner self must be examined and self-awareness raised. Awareness recovery means to raise your consciousness. Change must come from within. Recovery is an inside job.

What you want to achieve is what we call a good, happy life. Good and happy require various degrees of comfort and leisure, work, and play. This requires a balanced lifestyle. A balanced lifestyle is not something alcoholics and addicts think about when drunk and stoned. Now, with mental clarity available, it is something you can take seriously. A life balanced with worthwhile activities and aspirations becomes a nurtured and contented one.

M. Scott Peck, M.D., wrote in The Road Less Traveled, "A life of total dedication to the truth also means a life of willingness to be personally challenged." Accept any challenge that faces you and you will be surprised when you come to enjoy the new challenge.

What will be done with all the hours you suddenly have available each week? You need to use time constructively. Get creative in your future plans.

Give this a lot of thought. This should be carefully considered before leaving rehab. The sooner you start the better, because the details need consideration. The first idea is not always the best one, right? All those hours of wasted time that you once spent craving, obsessing, acquiring, using, and then entering mindless oblivion need to be filled. That time is precious now, isn't it? You can't get that time back, but you can use the time in the future.

In sobriety, any goal can be attained. A clear mind and a healthy body will make it so much easier to complete personal objectives for career, education, family life, and creative passions.

When reading this book, think of what you want to do in life. Take notes. Research the things that are of interest. Freedom from daily drinking and drugging means the mind is free to imagine a life grounded in reality.

Establishing beliefs, setting goals, maintaining clarity of mind and body, raising consciousness, and controlling your mind will be major areas emphasized throughout this book.

Reading Awareness Recovery will challenge you to raise your consciousness.

1. Discover You (True Self)

2. Know What You Believe

3. Establish Future Goals

4. Live a Balanced Life

5. Develop and Implement a Personal Exit Strategy

6. Increase Awareness of Being in the Now

7. Live Life Sober and Free

MATERIALS RECOMMENDED FOR EXIT
STRATEGY PLANNING:

- dictionary (don't skip over an unfamiliar word)

- black or blue pen

- colored felt highlighter

- one or two notebook(s) - this/these will be your
  exit strategy planner(s)

Write across the cover or on the spine of your notebook
"Exit Strategy" and your name, showing ownership and
expressing conviction and determination to escape the past
and welcome the future of personal freedom.

Establish a place where the rush and noisy madness of
society is absent, where you can be quiet and still and think.
Somewhere, you can be alone in silent solitude to contemplate
choices.

Somewhere that is sacred: a personal sanctuary. Go there
often. The benefits of silence cannot be overstated.

Hey Genius, Now What?

"When I was five years old, my mother always told me that happiness was the key to life. When I went to school, they asked me what I wanted to be when I grew up. I wrote down 'happy.' They told me I didn't understand the assignment, and I told them they didn't understand life."

JOHN LENNON, singer and songwriter

PONDERING THE PAST IS A great way to escape facing the future: it leads nowhere fast.

The difference between us and the non-addicted people of the world is only that we cannot enjoy an alcoholic drink at a celebration for New Year's or a birthday and forget about having a drink the next day. We could not have a line or three of cocaine with that drink and then not think about it again.

We wanted more. We became obsessed and addicted. Mentally and physically, we were attached to a substance that did us no good whatsoever and was detrimental to life. Acknowledge this and maybe you can change your mind.

We must change our beliefs to stop killing ourselves spiritually. We must have a change in consciousness to change our belief that drugs are good. This requires that we open our minds to new ideas, no matter where they come from. We need to be open to the new and different.

Hopefully, you are in a good place now. Feeling secure and unafraid of being open to a good life -which scares many; we seem to like fearing what lies ahead. The real positive stuff life can offer is freeing. How do we get there?

Forget fear. You will have an exit strategy.

Now, you will be consciously alert and feeling uplifted. You will find the way you used to be hard to believe, imagining how, on any given day at a moment like now, your mind would have been obsessing about the next shot, hit, and high. What a difference time makes when you spend it being focused on

15

good old-fashioned positive energy.

My perception has changed about life, and with it, many beliefs.

Here is a story about perception.

The young woman seated beside me in the public library was looking intently at her computer monitor. I was also looking at mine. I muttered, "Damn it!" I apologized to her and justified my curse by saying, "Sometimes these machines don't do as they are told." She reminded me that computers are slower than we'd like sometimes. I paused, relaxed, and took a deep breath.

"Thanks for reminding me." I knew she was right. It was true. After all, it was a public PC. Taking a deep breath again, I proceeded with my work.

Without any prompting from me, the young lady said, "I am looking at my astrology for December. It says there will be opportunities coming my way." She paused and then said, "There are some challenges too."

Clearly, she liked opportunities and saw them as good: positive situations to come. And it was also clear that she saw challenges as negative and possibly troubling: circumstances to overcome.

I turned to face her and said, "The opportunity that comes may be challenging. And the challenge might be in accepting the opportunity." She stopped scrolling and looked directly at me. When our eyes met, I offered an example.

"The opportunity might be that your dream job is offered, but it is in another country, and the challenge is to leave your life here and the family and friends that you cherish." I paused.

Her expression indicated she was considering what I had shared. She asked, "You think?"

I tried to clarify. "You might find it challenging to teach full-time at a high school in another state, but the opportunity to be a full-time teacher is exactly what you want."

Not sure, she asked, "So, the challenges can be a good thing for me next month?"

"The opportunity may come, and the challenge is only to accept it." I logged off my computer while she mulled over my comments. "Life gives you a challenge when you are ready for personal, spiritual, or intellectual growth."

I stood and put on my coat. Before I walked away, she said, "Thank you."

This story is easy for a genius like you to understand.

Looking on the bright side and being positive offers a more enlightening, open-minded perspective. It is the story of one word having a negative connotation. In this case, the word was challenge. I encouraged this woman to embrace a challenge as an opportunity. I left her with the idea that the challenge is there because she is ready for growth, for a new adventure.

Are you facing a challenge now? Can you see the opportunity that the challenge offers?

Being the genius you are, certainly you do. Will you be generous, kind, and loving to yourself?

Will benevolence guide your own spirit and be the consoling voice and healing force needed now within you?

Yes, I called you a genius. You are a genius to be where you are. You are safe. Somehow you figured out how to survive the challenges in life this far despite yourself. How fortuitous. Be grateful for that gift. In fact, that is why this book is specifically for you. There are many questions for you to contemplate and answer to help you plan for life after rehab. And you are smart enough to conceive an exit strategy with a little guidance.

Now is the most important and now is all that matters. The energy, thoughts, and feelings you have now can be negative or positive and will attract either bad and harmful people and results or good and healthful people and results.

You are where you are supposed to be. How do I know this? I know this because right now, you are where you are. The fact that you are reading this book means that is exactly what you are supposed to be doing at this moment in time. You can be grateful now for many things.

You had genius enough to get into a rehab instead of many more dreadful places. You are in a great place. Think about it. Look where you are now. Really, pause right now and look around you. Is everything okay? I mean right now, at this moment, are you safe? Are you in danger? Are you starving? Do you feel like complaining? What about?

If there is anything wrong, if you are distracted or worried about something, maybe you should set this book aside for a better time. When you are ready to focus on life after rehab, pick the book back up. Maybe there is a more appropriate time for you to begin thinking about what you will do after rehab.

If all is well, and you are comfortable and focused, then this is a good time.

You are in a great place in rehab. You could be in federal or state prison, county or city jail, the hospital ICU, a mental hospital, housed in a home for the physically impaired, waiting to die in a hospice, on probation while broke, angry, and hungry while wearing an ankle monitor, or homeless - but then again you could be a body in a morgue because of accidental death, murder, or suicide, or just be missing because you got lost: lost your mind.

The professionals at the treatment center are there to help you succeed.

You are a genius! You got into a rehab. You are in the right place at the right time and exactly where you are supposed to be. That is why you are where you are. What a great place to be! A place dedicated to helping you become better. You are reading a copy of Awareness Recovery to make plans for your future: a life of awareness recovery after rehab.

That's brilliant!

Right now, you may be only thinking about getting through today and each day following without your craving and obsession to drug and or drink driving you bonkers, cuckoo-nuts. But your mind will eventually clear. The craving will cease, vanish, evaporate into the ether. And you will be relieved and will feel grateful when you sense the drug obsession has been lifted. When you mind clears, you will see the future. The future is inevitable.

Only a fool tries to evade the inevitable. You are no fool. You know a future awaits you. The future will arrive. It is not predictable, nor is it foreseeable, but it can be shaped. Plans that are made and actions taken today will always determine and shape tomorrow.

Every genius knows that the saying "failing to plan is planning to fail" is true. You will begin planning a future after rehab by developing an exit strategy. An exit strategy is a roadmap for a life plan. What your ambitions, goals, and objectives will be.

Your goals or objectives, whichever word you prefer, need not be lofty, like "I will be an airline pilot in one year." The objective may be as simple as "I will begin to pay my bills on time," or "Next year, at this time, I will be out of debt and have started to save or invest my earnings." Or "I will be home when my children go to school in the morning and meet them when they come home every day."

How you will live life sober is your choice.

Write five goals in your exit strategy journal.

Then, write five things you can do each day to achieve each of the goals you have written.

Now commit yourself fully and follow though thoroughly. Here's an example.

Goal One: I will remain sober each day from now going forward, planning a future after rehab by developing an exit strategy. An exit strategy is a roadmap for a life plan. What your ambitions, goals, and objectives will be.

Your goals or objectives, whichever word you prefer, need not be lofty, like "I will be an airline pilot in one year." The objective may be as simple as "I will begin to pay my bills on time," or "Next year, at this time, I will be out of debt and have started to save or invest my earnings." Or "I will be home when my children go to school in the morning and meet them when they come home every day."

How you will live life sober is your choice.

Write five goals in your exit strategy journal.

Then, write five things you can do each day to achieve each of the goals you have written.

Now commit yourself fully and follow though thoroughly. Here's an example.

Goal One: I will remain sober each day from now going forward, you have already been released, it is not too late to get your sober future planned.

Living in sobriety really is the act of loving yourself. You will love being sober. Now you can love the future with enthusiasm, too. Love that you have a future. You are surely a genius to have figured out how to save enough of your life to have a chance to love and live free again. Free of drugs and free from pain and free from self-destructive behavior.

Getting started planning makes you smart, and courageous too.

Can you see a future now? Make that future sacred to you. Cherish it and live today to fulfill tomorrow's promise. The future for you can hold happiness. Love waits there, too. As you love yourself, others will love you. Healing has begun.

Begin a journey about love.

Start by learning to love you. Love is the key to successful and positive healing and growth. It does not take a genius to know this, but you are a genius, so it should be obvious to you. Life is successful and complete with love. Love is the key to freedom that unlocks and opens your heart and mind. "All you need is love," wrote the songwriter John Lennon.

He was serious.

The fine arts and literary culture of our society refer to Lennon as a genius. Like you, he lived influenced by drug abuse. He overcame that. You can, too. Lennon quit harming himself. You can, too. Every genius knows that love is an essential human need.

All you need is love, and to love, you need to love yourself first. You must find a way to love you. You must become someone you love. Let nothing and no one prevent that healing. A great man once said, "Love thy neighbor as you would yourself." The question clearly is, how can you love your neighbor if you do not love you?

Picture, you as you would really like to be.

Is that image of you someone you can love? Did you imagine yourself, beautiful and rich? Did you conjure a vain, arrogant, and pompous person? Is that someone you could love?

Indulge yourself now. Go back in time in your mind. Go back, as far back as you can, in your mind's memory. Remember a young you. Remember that child now. Remember when you were innocent? It was a long time ago. Picture innocent you.

Now, think about a happy time. Remember a smile and laughter and excitement about something. Think of a time when you knew love. Do you recall anyone who loved you? Bring back the memory of that person. You loved them.

The self that you find in the memories of your mind will reveal an image of love that can be held sacred. That child you were is loveable. Love that one. Love is sacred. Give love to that sacred you because you are your inner self.

The inner you consist of your mind-soul-psyche (MSP). The dictionary defines the mind as the psyche and the psyche as the soul. This is your consciousness. It is the inner you that you will heal through your own efforts. You will grow physically well and become spiritually evolved and intellectually competent and maybe inspired.

This is the soul's sole purpose.

Beyond the Influence, by Katherine Ketcham and William F. Asbury, includes symptoms published by the American Psychiatric Associations in the Di-agnostic and Statistical Manual of Mental Disorders (DSM-IV) - here is a review of what it takes to be an alcohol addict.

1. Tolerance

2. Withdrawal symptoms, which include hand tremors, sweating, elevated pulse rate, insomnia, nausea, or anxiety; these symptoms may develop into hallucinations, seizures, and/or psychotic symptoms

3. Drinking larger amounts over longer periods than intended

4. Persistent desire or unsuccessful attempts to cut down or control drinking

5. Spending a significant amount of time trying to obtain alcohol, drink alcohol, or recover from its effects

6. Giving up social, occupational, or recreational activities because of alcohol

7. Continuing to drink despite persistent or recurrent physical or psychological problems caused or exacerbated by alcohol use

Problem drinking is also described in the DSM-IV as 1) problems resulting at work, school, or home; 2) situations that put your life or other people's lives at risk; 3) legal problems like driving citations and arrests; 4) interpersonal problems, such as arguments with family and friends, barroom brawls, and other physical confrontations.

Replace the word alcohol with anything you have a problem controlling, from cocaine or Vicodin to gambling, and if three or more of these symptoms clearly and honestly exist or are conspicuous to others, and you are in rehab or incarcerated, then keep reading, because you may have an addiction problem. You may really want an exit strategy of your own.

Rehab, recovery, and relapse is a discouraging cycle. Neither treatment centers for substance abuse nor correctional facilities succeed in sufficient rehabilitation to stop most users from abusing. Ending addiction to alcohol and drugs requires your full commitment. You must decide to do no harm. You must decide to love yourself.

Drug-free living brings clarity of mind and a clear conscience. Living in such a manner can only bring a productive and a trouble-free life. Of course, there will be challenges and difficulties, but sober, you can address the problem instead of drinking and sinking to drown, or doping and hoping life goes away.

Now go back and read, if you did not, the Preface and the Introduction to this book. There is information there that you need to proceed successfully through the entire book. You must be thorough in designing a doable exit strategy.

It is crucial that from here forward, you act with maximum integrity and determination in your everyday routine. You are going to be the hero of this new chapter in your life. Heroes make mistakes but they don't stop when they meet adversity. Nothing stops them from jumping hurdles and moving roadblocks as they pursue their destination, fulfilling their destiny.

Take a moment and write your beliefs about each of the following controversial subjects. This is a good way to examine if what you think you believe is still relevant.

1. Your religion

2. Other religions

3. Your political viewpoint

4. Social values (abortion, gay marriage, death penalty)

5. Race relations and ethnic biases

6. Gender (equality, disparity)

7. Class differences (the wealthy versus middle class vs the poor)

8. Money

9. Relationships (intimate, friendships, coworkers, employers)

10. Weight and issues or concerns on the subject

11. Homelessness

12. Guns and gun control

Take time to really think about how strong your beliefs are about each of these twelve topics. Then consider what could be changed and reconsidered. For instance, there was a time when I was strongly opposed to the death penalty. I revised my belief that the death penalty should be abolished after working in the prison system and learning of the atrocities some men had committed. In one case, a man had gone on a killing spree and, in one weekend, killed eleven people. He was given eleven life sentences. Is that better than a death sentence?

Explore what convictions you have now and revisit these statements again to see if anything has changed during sobriety.

Expanding beliefs with a mind open to new ideas and perspectives increases our own awareness.

You Crazy You

"Dying ain't much of a living."

THE OUTLAW JOSEY WALES is a character in the movie with the same name.

YES, YOU ARE CRAZY. SOMETIMES you know it, and sometimes you will acknowledge it but still won't accept it. Not accepting you have a problem with substance abuse only makes you crazier. You are crazy enough to believe that no one can tell that you are under the influence of something. The reality is that everyone can tell. They simply accept you because they are also under the influence, or accepting of your intoxication because you are maintaining control of your speech and motor skills.

The belief that no one knows you are high except you is what makes you crazy, but it does not diminish your unique genius. It is okay to believe still that you have a unique genius. Not with arrogance, but with confidence. Still, believe that you have courage and are strong. Not with self-importance and conceit, but modesty and humility.

A person can be a crazy genius.

You are not all that different. As smart as you are, your sanity is questionable because you drank, smoked, snorted, shot-up, bumped, and popped pills and any substance you could get your hands on to change the way you felt. That was crazy. You did not like the way you felt or the thoughts that were in your mind, so you altered your mind with substances to the extent that even you could see the fringe of lunacy. You questioned your own sanity at times. Or someone told you, "You're crazy!"

Once you get rid of the drug habit, you will be able to tap into your true genius. Life will get better.

You will learn to deal with reality and respond to the world rationally and responsibly, accepting life as a mature adult.

Reality was so unbearable because you had issues with life as it is. Instead of seeking legitimate help, you dosed yourself up with all the drugs you could. That was not genius. That was fear.

Learning anything requires research and thorough comprehension of what is being studied. Get a dictionary. This book is not for a counselor, therapist, or sponsor to decipher and explain to you. This is for you to increase your knowledge about the way to live without drugging and drinking yourself to death: slow suicide.

Get free. Free your mind with education. Escape the possibility of forever being pitied by your family, by the courts employers, and business associates. Show the world how a real genius operates.

It does not get any more real than where you are right now. Real life is happening now, so what would you like most to happen? Many people in treatment want to be free of the entire rehab situation. They don't like it. It wasn't their decision. It was an intervention by family or spouse or maybe even court ordered. They want to get back to doing what they were doing before this treatment-center nonsense came along. If that is you and you have a hard copy of this book, give it away to someone who wants to save their life.

Few clients/patients in treatment facilities embrace fully the help being offered to them. They reject it the way a three-year-old child rejects eating vegetables. This is very ineffective and immature.

You want to do the opposite. If you want to be free of the situation, the solution is acceptance.

Accept that you have a problem and follow counseling and medical instructions. This will change the situation of rehab in a productive and positive way. Accepting your addiction and accepting help with enthusiasm will make every moment in rehab a joy. That will free you of the stress, anxiety, self-pity, and anger.

Gary Zukav, author of The Seat of the Soul, writes, "You cannot begin the work of releasing an addiction until you can acknowledge that you are addicted." He explains further that "Acknowledging an addiction, accepting that you have an addiction, is acknowledgment that a part of you is out of control." And "Once an addiction has been acknowledged, it cannot be ignored, and it cannot be released without changing your life, without changing your self-image, without changing your entire perceptual and conceptual framework. We do not want to do that because it is our nature to resist change."

Resistance to change is especially deeply rooted in those with addictions. That is why the addict is an addict.

To get and stay and be free now, you should do what you do not want to do. Remember that doing what you want has gotten you where you are now.

You will grow from acceptance of the situation into excitement about learning and then move into enthusiasm about the new life ahead.

What does freedom mean to you? The first thing that comes to mind is to be free to do as you please. Doing what you please led you on a self-destructive journey. If you change your desires to life-supporting ambitions to achieve productive goals, there will be a dynamic shift in the direction your life flows.

All you are going to do is change your perception enough to choose positively instead of negatively. It is not that hard, because you already know what the negative choices are and the results they bring. When the crack dealer calls, hang up. He's not your friend. Find an alcohol-free coffee house, make friends there, and leave the sports-bar scene. Identifying dark forces as harmful and immediately turning away to face the light, even running to the source of light, will bring the right results every time. Practice this, and soon, your true genius will be apparent to all. No harm will be done, and you will have no regrets.

Better living comes with acknowledging and accepting the truth. Being honest with yourself will allow you to make nondestructive decisions and take harmless actions.

If you are on your way to rehabilitation treatment or currently in rehab for substance abuse and chemical dependency, then you have been living on the road to ruin. A life directed by self-will and desire for instant self-gratification results in cheap thrills. These thrills do not fulfill your life purpose. Hasty, impulsive decisions driven by a desire to feel good are characteristic of an addict.

Someone could have an addiction to sugar and need a milkshake every day or a box of cookies every night. Some sugar junkies are also caffeine addicts. They start with a Coca-Cola first thing in the morning. The sugar and caffeine addicts will ruin their health but not their entire life.

As your mind clears, you will recognize dark forces. Then, by slowing down to live in the moment, you will have the time to evaluate each opportunity for its value. You will pause and consider whether the opportunity that has presented itself is good or bad. Instead of the impulsive, drug-addled, and alcohol-soaked mind driving your decisions, you will, with a clear mind, give yourself time to think. Does that make sense?

Getting free is the first step at this point. Freeing yourself from self-harm comes first, and to do this, irrational thinking must end. What we want to be free from must be very clear in our mind. Write down a list of people and, places, and things to eliminate from your life. And list the behaviors that you do not want to keep.

Of course, your favorite drugs will be listed under things. Other things might be free of self-importance? Rid of narcissm? Free of bad habits? Free of over-indulgence? Stop being judgmental of people that you do not even know? Maybe one of these strikes a chord for you. Consider things that people have told you about yourself that you disputed, like when someone said, "You're a liar!"

It is important to grasp your smallness in the big scheme of things. You have little authority. But you are not an infant without any authority at all. Recognize what you can control and what you cannot control. This is something mature adults distinguish daily in the context of their personal, professional, and social life.

You exhibit a lack of maturity that does not allow your true genius to be seen when you fail to acknowledge your strengths, weaknesses, and limitations. Because you have been unsuccessful at ruling the world, you leaned on alcohol or drugs to create an illusion of the world more to your liking. Awareness recovery will bring a more realistic worldview. Raising your awareness will raise your ability to shine.

Freeing yourself from bad habits requires you identify your bad habits. What do you want to change to improve your ability to function successfully in society?

There are many habits that people have that are bad. Make your own list in your journal. Here are a few examples, just to start your imagination going.

1. Spitting in public

2. Biting fingernails

3. Bragging

4. Saying "um" between words

5. Talking loudly or too softly (do people have to tell you to lower your voice or to speak louder often?)

6. Chewing with your mouth open

7. Talking with your hands

8. Using curse words in every sentence

List the bad habits that you have today in your exit strategy journal.

This is a start. Begin working to stop these self-acknowledged bad habits.

By writing them down, your mind has placed these behaviors in the "do not do" column. These are bad habits you know about yourself. No one had to tell you they are bad. You already knew that. Often it is that you know right from wrong and yet think it cool. You already knew drugging and popping pills was bad, yet you did it. You already knew vodka for breakfast was bad, yet you did it. The behaviors that you listed above are the same. You know better, yet you do them.

These are bad habits because you do them impulsively and even compulsively (without thinking). It is not that you are ignorant of how offensive the behavior is. You convinced yourself it was cool to walk like Al Pacino in the movie Scarface.

Now that you have identified behaviors that you want to eliminate, your mind will help you and, catch you and redirect you.

You will hear yourself about to curse to describe something when talking, and...you will hear it happening and...STOP. You will see yourself about to use your hands to describe something when talking and...you will see it happening and...STOP. You will be aware of what you are doing when you are doing the action.

This is awareness recovery in action.

Here is an example of three men completely unaware of reality, and so their bad decisions produce actions that suck. Their awareness is so low they are incapable of rational thought.

The Three Stooges were a comedy team in early American film and television. In one episode, all three of them are on a rowboat in a lake. The rowboat springs a leak. The boat begins filling up with water. The three men panic. What to do? Moe shouts, "Let the water out!" Curly takes an oar and bashes a hole in the bottom of the boat to let the water out! And they stand surprised until Moe demands, "Get a bucket!" And they begin bailing the water out of the boat with a bucket.

It was funny. We like to laugh at stupid.

Making a hole in the bottom of the boat to let the water out is crazy, right? Not much genius, though. Isn't this the kind of decision-making that happens on booze and drugs? What to do? Hide the bottle!

Flush the dope!

One saying widely repeated amongst people in recovery programs is, "The definition of insanity is doing the same thing over and over and expecting different results."

Thinking irrationally and then acting irrationally, being incapable of foreseeing the likely sad consequences, and then doing the same thing again, is insane. This is what happens when we lose touch with reality. A clear mind will, when freed from mind-altering substances, stay in touch with reality. Then, your true genius and clear mind will be apparent to everyone you meet.

My drinking at one time became so habitual, it was normal. Saturday night keg parties were regular occurrences in high school, and Sunday afternoon football games required beer. When I began work, drinking after work with co-workers was perfectly normal. Then, drinking a Scotch on the rocks alone after work became a nightly ritual. Then, twenty-plus years later, I was drinking vodka screwdrivers or margaritas for Sunday's breakfast. It was normal. It was my norm. It was normal to me and the alcoholic women in my life.

Eventually, this normal behavior led to an alcohol rehabilitation program. I had to get humble.

Fortunately, I had the capacity to do this.

Accepting the humiliating situation, I found myself in, and that it was the result of my own actions, wasn't easy, but it was necessary to become willing and open to receive help.

Many residential clients/patients rebel in childish belligerence. They don't like the group counseling, they don't like the food, and they choose a movie anytime over a spiritual mentoring workshop.

When I entered rehab, I was mature enough to see my folly was destructive and turned my focus on accepting help and guidance.

Others during my inpatient stay were not ready to admit their own reckless folly. They were plainly in denial. They just wanted to play what they called the game, but I did not see a game. I saw that my life had crumbled.

And that if I was any type of genius, then I had better use my full mind and take full advantage of this rehab opportunity.

It doesn't take much genius to grab the rope when sinking in quicksand. How deep is one's denial? Is one going to say, "No, I knew it was quicksand, there! I just wanted to see how deep it is! I will let you know when I reach the bottom!"

In the country song "View from the Bottom," Dude Mowry warns, "If you're not happy at the top, don't stop on the road to ruin. Chase the women; drink the whisky; smoke 'em if you got 'em. Here's a postcard from hell. It's a view from the bottom."

Being honest and opening my mind to the ideas presented by sober people and people without addiction to alcohol worked for me. It was a wise decision. This increased my chances of getting sober and improving my life. Being spiritually and mentally free was desirable. I had to maintain an open mind and accept that learning new behavior was critical. An open mind works for everyone, and it will work for you, too.

Once you are in the hole, you are already at the bot-tom. I had dug myself into a hole full of booze, and I required help to get out. I had hit bottom. There isn't anything to be proud of, and no one can get out of it by denying the mess they are in.

This is what you want to avoid happening as you begin life after rehab. Stepping into another hole on the way out the door is not a requirement. Having a plan of action and an exit strategy that details what you will do after rehab to stay sober will be an enormous help.

Free your mind. Free it of the notion that you have a clue what to do. Suspend the belief that you know something. Open your mind; make it like an empty bucket waiting to be filled. Clear you mind. Make it as a dry sponge waiting to absorb knowledge. All your best thinking got you a front-row seat in a rehab for substance abuse. Drop the pretense of a know-it-all. Accept your need to learn not to stumble, trip, and fall when you walk. It doesn't take a genius to walk straight. You've got enough genius to just do it.

When told not to put your hand on a hot stove, why do you? "Don't drink too much," people warn. "But how much is too much?" questions the alcoholic. "Don't put that needle in your arm," people warn. "It will kill you." "But how will I know if I don't try?" questions the junkie.

No one held a gun to your head and made you light that stem. No one tied you down and shot the dope up your vein. No one put six prescription pills in your mouth and rubbed your throat till you swallowed.

You will learn in rehab what you missed in kindergarten.

You did not go to kindergarten? Welcome, then! Let's start at day one. Lesson number one is to be honest and always tell the truth. Lesson number two is to do no harm. That's it for day one. That will begin increasing your awareness.

And don't forget your bad-habits list. Writing things down by hand with pen and paper helps your mind remember what not to forget.

As we proceed, you will continuously be recovering awareness. This means regaining control of your mind. By doing so, you will know what you are thinking before you do something without think-ing. That's the first sure way to show off your natural genius.

Napoleon Hill, author of Think and Grow Rich, states, "Our only limitations are those we set up in our own minds."

If you have not been paying attention so far, start paying attention to the help offered to you.

Listen to what is being said. Reflect on it. Start the practice of being fully present and attentive in every situation instead of daydreaming. Be there now.

Someone is speaking to you. What did they say?

Ask them to repeat the information when they pause, but don't interrupt. Wait. Be courteous. Often, someone else may also need the information repeated as well. You will always learn more prac-ticing patience and attentiveness.

The more you disagree with information presented to you, the more likely that it is exactly what you need to pay the most attention to. When an idea rubs you the wrong way, it is likely to be hitting close to home, to be true. Get your mind to thinking about what is going on inside you.

If you remain always in your comfort zone mentally and emotionally, and are never challenged, then growth will not occur. There will be no change in you, and that means no spiritual or intellectual growth. You will remain mostly ignorant of the most important person on the planet: YOU.

The time you have in rehabilitation should be perceived as a blessing or gift: a positive reprieve from your active self-destruction. You do not want to leave the treatment center empty-handed, with zilch. Bring zeal and zest to each day's activity. Be prepared for meetings with your counselor.

Once acceptance of your reality and of the seriousness of your addiction is established, it will be easier to become enthusiastic about the rehabilitation process. You are saving your life. It may even become exciting to love yourself.

If you remain ashamed of being in rehab, you will remain downhearted. Depression is likely to set in. Now you have another problem. Depression is toxic to your spiritual consciousness. Positive thinking about this experience will keep you feeling good emotionally.

Remember, a wasted mind is never wanted.

Beginning a new lifestyle is better than accepting a stalemate. A stalemate occurs when you hold on to the past, reject the present, and are fearful of the future. Life offers no stalemate. It is do or be done. Win or lose - and you can be a winner. Free yourself from the past. Live in the now and enjoy the moment.

Facing Fact

"You gotta keep changing. Shirts, old ladies, whatever.

I'd rather keep changing and lose a lot of people along the way. If that's the price, I'll pay it."

NEIL YOUNG, singer and songwriter

THE CHALLENGE FOR YOU IS TO CHANGE your conscious-ness.

Your mind has done you a disservice somewhere along the way. You lost control of your sane mind, but it was always your mind to lose. That's the only honest way to assess your being in a rehab or a jail or a hospital's Intensive Care Unit. Use your genius now to re-train your mind to serve you to its best ability. It is your mind. Your mind is your own. Own it. Control it.

Learn something with your body and your mind learns how to do it as well. For instance, rowing a boat requires that you row the boat physically, and then your mind understands, and you can say, "I already know how to roll a boat" because you have actually done it. Bowling is the same. Basketball is, too. There is no way to learn karate just by reading about it. Knitting, bicycling, and most physical activities must be done to be learned. And they become either a habit or a natural reflexive action.

What you will learn is the idea that action can change your mind just as much as your mind can change your actions and behavior. You will lose bad habits by practicing new habits that you believe will be beneficial to you.

In preparing an exit strategy, you want to include daily activities. Educating yourself positively, challenging yourself with new healthy experiences, and accomplishing objectives are the keys to a happy, sober life.

For instance, let us assume that you have a habit of brushing your teeth in the morning. And when you do not, you feel uncomfortable until you do. Now suppose you choose as part of your daily sober living habits to brush your teeth before you go to sleep. You begin practicing this new habit for a month, and soon, you will not feel comfortable sleeping until you brush your teeth.

Soon, you will believe that brushing your teeth in the evening is a good idea. It makes sense to clean your mouth and teeth, removing all the debris of food and sugary drinks you have put in your mouth throughout the day. After a few weeks, brushing your teeth before bedtime becomes a habit. By performing the action, you have altered your mindset.

You could do the same thing with showering and bathing. You could come to believe that at the end of a sober day, it makes sense to take off your dirty clothes instead of passing out in them on the couch. End the day by showering or bathing and washing all the day's dirt off before going to a clean bed.

These are the types of things that will be suggested throughout this book. The idea is that you take notes and highlight sections that interest you so you build an exit strategy for staying sober after rehab. There are many options. Keep an open mind. Be courageous. Try things you have not done before. Begin to accept responsibility for your own mind, body, and soul. That is the way a drug-free genius operates. Sober.

Remember the Alamo! Have you heard that call to arms? It was the battle cry of the men who fought under the command of General Sam Houston (1793-1863) in the battle won by the Texans at San Jacinto.

Houston was a heavy drinker. His alcoholism was a topic for gossip. Still, Houston was a brilliant military leader.

Houston ordered the attack at San Jacinto in April 1836. The victory proved decisive and secured Texas its independence.

But as far as the Alamo story, Houston had ordered the fort called the Alamo in San Antonio, Texas to be deserted and destroyed in 1835. He had determined it could not be defended successfully in the war Texas was fighting against Mexico.

He sent Colonel James Bowie (1796-1836), already known for his famous "Bowie knife," to carry out the orders. The orders were to destroy Fort Alamo so nothing would be left for the Mexican armies to seize. Bowie defied these orders.

Colonel James Bowie, upon arriving at the Alamo with its volunteer Texan fighting men, decided to defend the fort in contradiction to General Sam Houston's orders. What was he thinking? (Was he drinking too?) It is clear he challenged and resisted authority.

Bowie never gathered more than 142 fighting men at the Alamo, even though they kept sending couriered messages to Colonel Fannin in Goliad to requesting reinforcements.

Colonel Bowie shared command with Colonel Travis. Soon, they were joined by several men from Tennessee, led by David Crockett. None of them considered getting out of there, as General Houston had ordered. They never considered an exit strategy.

General Antonio López de Santa Anna marched 5,500 hundred troops from the Rio Grande to San Antonio in six days. On March 6, 1836, the Alamo was lost by the Texans in a merciless slaughter. No one was spared. Details of this battle are well chronicled.

That same year, 1836, Sam Houston was elected the first president of the republic of Texas.

Like James Bowie, many people are delusional about their capabilities. Their time and energy is too precious to be compromised by the insight of anyone else. They will not give up a fight. Why James Bowie thought Fort Alamo was worth salvaging and that he could do it with 142 men, no one will ever know. It could have been pride, and it could have been whiskey, or the combination of the two. The responsible thing for Bowie to do when he arrived at the Alamo was to follow instructions: the orders General Houston had given.

Many people are self-centered. They believe they must come first, be first, and that others should cater to their whims. Selfishness and self-centered-ness are common traits in addicts. If you find this true of yourself, find a way to correct this, because it is a character trait that will result in frustration and unhappiness. Being self-serving is frequently self-defeating. Dissatisfaction plagues every day.

Nothing is good enough for you. Because, you believe you are not worthy to receive what is offered. This is the result of low self-esteem a lack of self-respect.

Once you become more giving, a transformation takes place that allows you to receive with gratitude. You will earnestly say, "Thank you so much." And people will see you are open to receive, and when you reciprocate and give back generously, other people will say thank you in appreciation of the smallest thing you offer. This type of relationship is likely to be suspicious to you if you have much experience within selfish social circles.

When you work with open and generous social interactions and take to heart loving and charitable relations, then you may come to believe that giving is better than receiving.

When practicing random acts of kindness, I looked for ways I could make a person smile, and for a moment, they would have a bright spot in their day. Simply saying, "You are very efficient," to a cashier or a bank teller makes them feel appreciated, regardless of what troubles they are having. People like to be appreciated. And people will appreciate your compliment or assistance.

Whenever you feel something is wrong, it is likely that something is wrong, but look inside yourself first. Check yourself before you wreck yourself.

This can be done in subtle circumstances as well as in traumatic situations. Maybe being late for an appointment, class, or work makes you frustrated when something or someone slows you down, and you have to squelch your urge to shout, "Hurry up!" to the server, bringing your iced caramel macchiato. You took the time to order even though it would make you later than you already are - but you have to have your iced caramel macchiato. After all, you should have what you want when you want it.

Young people are always in a rush. No one knows why. They usually drive fast and are still hardly ever on time. They eat fast, talk fast, and very often don't hear a word anyone else says. All that behavior is due to self-centered character traits.

I rear-ended a car at age nineteen. Hurrying to get on the highway, I saw an opening and hit the gas before making sure the driver in front of me had moved into traffic. Decades later, I was the older driver waiting for an opening to merge into when I saw, in my driver's side mirror, a car only seconds before it rear-ended me. The driver of that car was nineteen and she was in a hurry to get to work at Taco Bell two blocks away. At nineteen, each of us was only focused on our need to get somewhere fast. It didn't work for either of us. Focused so intently on our rush, we ignored what was really going on ahead of us. A man once boasted that he had never stolen anything.

I asked him, "What about the time you stole from your wife while you spent all afternoon drinking with your friends?"

He came to realize that he had stolen time from his family in his selfish addiction behavior of drinking from the time he got off work until he passed out on the couch at home. And the weekends were for him to unwind. That meant a more inebriated state of mind.

No time spent reading to the children, or listening to his wife's concerns, because he was working and tired and needed to relax first. His form of relaxation did not nurture love within his family. He had stolen family time.

Things happen in life that are beyond our control. Being hit in the rear by another car is very rarely your fault, unless you slammed on the brakes suddenly to avoid a squirrel. Take away the squirrel. When a car hits you from behind, it is that driver's fault. You know that is true at once.

But when you get out of the car, the driver that rear-ended you is mad and blaming you for stopping at the light as it turned yellow. "You're supposed to speed up when it turns yellow!" he screams. "You made me spill my iced caramel macchiato!"

Whenever something feels wrong, it is likely true that something is wrong. What is wrong is most often wrong only to you. You are feeling there is something wrong. That is your intuition. Listen to your intuition when those moments happen. No one else can. Examine yourself before pointing fingers at someone else. Take your time. Be smart enough to look inside first and then assess what is going on around you. See if you have made a mistake. If so, or even if not, then acknowledge the situation and, most importantly, accept it.

Have you ever been bored? Are you finding it hard to accept the tedious lifestyle you have manifested? It is the boring person that says, "I am bored."

Think about that. It is true. Watching court TV programs and Jerry Springer reruns is boring. If that is what you are doing - you are boring.

Reality is what we make it. I am sure you have heard people say, "I am bored." We all have. I have said it. I don't anymore. I do not need to be bored being sober. My mind is clear. I can change what I am doing at any moment. Life with a clear mind is exciting, and I find myself with renewed enthusiasm for what I will accomplish in the morning and what lies ahead for the afternoon.

Drinking and drugging makes you more boring.

Sober life can be exciting because the mind is working, filled with imagination and fresh ideas! If you find a dull moment, as a sober person, all you must do is do something else. If the book you are reading becomes boring, go outside for a walk; if the walk is not interesting, go to a movie, or call a friend to go with you to a museum or the gym. Sober people have options. Their lives are not handicapped by mind-altering drink and drugs.

Have you ever realized that you need to go somewhere and meet someone, but you can't because you are too high? You start drinking or drugging at noon, and three hours later, you are intoxicated. There is no way you can meet with your spouse's parents for dinner, or, worse yet, with your probation officer.

What a gentle euphemism "altering" is in the phrase "mind-altering drugs." The truth is that the street drugs and prescriptions drugs you have abused are mind-stupefying. Not in any way mind-expanding, and in no way mind-enhancing.

Let's face the facts. Alcohol is a drug. Ethanol is the principal chemical found in alcoholic beverages. It is a psychoactive drug. There is no need to say anything about Vicodin, Xanax, heroin, cocaine, methamphetamine, hash, or marijuana, is there? Facing the facts sucks sometimes but always proves beneficial.

Facts are reality, and reality is made up of the truth.

Why is it so hard for some to face the facts: the truth?

Facing facts requires honesty. For the active alcoholic and addict, the truth is not a friend. The truth is cruel and unjust and only punishes and ruins a good buzz. "Truth or reality is avoided when it is painful," writes M. Scott Peck in The Road Less Traveled. He adds, "A life of total dedication to the truth also means a life of willingness to be personally challenged."

Substance abusers tend to be stubborn, non-conforming, belligerent, and self-centered.

These characteristics do not make it easy to be truthful or to face the changes reality brings. But you see that despite years spent denying the truth and avoiding reality, you have still been presented with the challenge of becoming a sober and productive member of society.

One man in a Twelve Step meeting shared plainly and truthfully, "I lied to get into 'it,' I lied to get out of 'it,' and I lied to keep the 'it' I lied to get."

Lying comes in many forms. There is no such thing as a white lie. A lie is a lie. Denial is lying to self. Living in denial of who we are and what suffering has been caused to ourselves and others is so much easier than facing facts. Deceit and deception are easier than facing a true reality. Until you get caught!

Do you have good character traits? Can you be honest even when it hurts? You don't steal much, do you? You stopped cheating when you got divorced, right? There are some good things about you.

None of these undesirable descriptions fit you: irresponsible, immature, unreliable, greedy, gluttonous, undisciplined, slothful, well-intentioned but manipulative, dishonest, deceitful, disloyal, devoid of prudence, financially reckless, pompous, vain. None of these adjectives describe you. Am I right?

You just like to drink and drug. That's all.

Now, you just have to stop drinking or drugging for a little while, and everything will be okay again. Any other problems will go away soon. They will vanish into the ether like air from a belch. All will be well.

Fact is that you should quit abusing booze and drugs. Didn't anyone tell you yet? You can't do either anymore, forevermore. That's the truth. No marijuana for the alcoholic. Brandy is not okay for the OxyContin or Vicodin addict.

You must quit getting high altogether.

Awareness recovery requires that your mind not be altered by a mind-altering chemical substance. You should want this for yourself.

Creating your own exit strategy will free you to have more of what you truly want in life.

If you want to avoid the possibilities of an early grave, insanity, homelessness, lengthy incarceration, and illness, then you will want to quit. The big question is: What will you do to get sober? Can you respect yourself enough to stop harming yourself? Do you care enough about life to stop harming others? What is your normal response to suggestions made to you? Do you follow advice well? When you come to a stop sign on the road, do you stop or drive slower? Can you be honest? Good. Be honest with yourself. You have a problem and you want to get rid of the problem by solving it. You want to learn a solution. You are ready to do anything to have a safe and happy life.

Honesty helps clear the mind. The soul feels better, too, and there's less stress on you.

Life is easier when you're not occupied with remembering lies. The inability to follow instructions and laws and policies and proper procedures - anyone's rules and regulations - was a shortcoming of my character in the past. I liked shortcuts, too. Then I learned that taking my time and doing it right the first time meant it didn't have to be paid for or done again.

The biggest fault many of us have is failure to follow instructions thoroughly.

Getting your mind in a condition capable of following instructions is the first objective.

Your mind gets in better shape simply by not getting high. Your mind gets in greater shape and strengthens when it is exercised. Makes sense, doesn't it? The drug-altered and - addled mind does not have the strength to even follow instructions, laws, or rules.

As your mind strengthens, sharpens, and clears, new ideas will come to you and different perspectives about what you have to deal with in life will emerge, be revealed. New insight will come in sudden bursts of intuition, and you will say to yourself, "Aha!"

Rebecca Rosen writes in her book Spirited, "The first challenge lies within you - you must learn to distinguish between a mind thought and an intuitive thought. A mind thought is a trailed thought, where you think of something, which leads to another thought, and another... Meanwhile, an intuitive thought just pops in from out of the blue, with nothing attached to it."

The mind-trail thought can get us lost as one thought leads to another and another. We might even forget the original thought. (That's why it helps to write things down.) When a great intuitive thought hits you, it strikes like a flash of lightning, so write it down immediately!

FOLLOW INSTRUCTIONS

If Jack had followed the law, he never would have found the AA Twelve Step program. "Then it was meant to be," Jack sighed. "Guess I missed the day at school when the teacher said we have to pay attention. And follow instructions."

Whenever we meticulously and carefully follow instructions, we get the results that the instructions provide. That is the key. Follow the verbal or written instructions of someone who knows more than you.

Alcoholics Anonymous suggests that you do the work required of the Twelve Steps. Those are the instructions: attend meetings, provide service to others, and pray and meditate daily. This is a way to achieve a sober life of contentment. Then, this is what must be done to achieve the results promised.

If you are told the way to get certain results and you want those results, then you must follow instructions. And you must follow the instructions with passionate desire and persistence because the results you have chosen to pursue are now a personal goal. To attain an objective and to accomplish a specific goal takes all your effort. Half measures will get you nowhere. As some of you have perhaps learned, if you do something half-assed you get half-assed results.

If you want to get the grade of A in a course of study, what do you have to do? In my own experience, the students that passed with A's were the ones who came to class earnestly, eager to be enlightened and educated, to learn something. They exhibited excitement and enthusiasm every day.

It turns out that achieving things is not that hard if you really want the results, put in the necessary effort, and follow the instructions. You know how it goes when you discard the instructions for a new tool or appliance before assembling or using it. Therefore, developing an exit strategy for rehab, jail, or even divorce, is critical.

The exit strategy that you finally choose is your instructions. Writing your own instructions while sober in rehab means that the instructions are likely to be realistic, possible, and attainable.

Here is an excerpt from a Fortune Builders publication, The Twelve Commandments of How Wealthy People Think: "Because of my own experience and my studies of other successful investors, I have come to realize that everything starts and ends in the mind."

Everything in your world of reality and influence begins and ends with your mind.

No Plan

"If you don't know where you are going, you might not get there."

YOGI BERRA, Professional baseball catcher, manager, and coach

A MIDDLE-AGED MAN TOLD ME his experience of leaving rehab. Tony had completed seven days in detox and thirty days in residential inpatient treatment.

During these thirty-seven days, he had been cooked for, housed, and kept on a schedule from seven in the morning until ten at night. The detox days had horrible results because he had been given drugs.

Once at the residences, Tony needed four days to get his head clear. When he did, he progressed quickly and happily. He enjoyed the diversity of counseling topics in group sessions, and the food was first-class, balanced, and organic, three meals a day.

During Tony's second week at the rehab, news came that a recently released patient had died from an overdose. Her name was Donna. She was nineteen years old, friendly, enthusiastic most days, curious, and full of energy. She was an intravenous drug user. Tony had met her while in treatment. They got along well together. Donna had used a lethal combination of meth and cocaine a week after release from rehab. Her mother had found her body in the basement of their suburban Maryland home. Sadness filled the hearts of many of the remaining rehab residents who had known Donna.

Tony then said that a man in his late thirties named Dave also died soon after release from the rehab. Dave had been given a ride to the airport by Mark, a long-term treatment resident who had earned driving privileges. Mark witnessed Dave order a drink at the airport bar lounge. Dave, like Donna, had been an intravenous drug user. He had only been away from the rehab for a week when he shot up the dope that his body could no longer handle. Yes, Dave had died.

Tony told me about the day he was released from treatment and left the rehab residences. He told me that he felt good that day, at least at first. He liked being sober again, even if it had only been thirty-seven days. The treatment center gave him an Alcoholics Anonymous thirty-day token and a certificate of program completion. Tony asked the administration if he could stay a few more days. He did not know where to go. He had made no plans for living life after release from rehab. The administration denied him further housing. Tony was looking at a homeless street life.

He got the hugs and handshakes after breakfast from his fellow addicts. All fifty or more got into the vans, just as he had for a month. And the vans left. He had never been at the residences during the morning hours of a day when there was treatment programming. There was one staff member there. There were no landline phones. There were no telephone books. He stood in the courtyard with his luggage and felt lonely. Tony even felt abandoned, but that got confused with feelings of rejection.

Tony told me that he did not know anything about North Miami. All he knew was the other patients, the residences, the programming building, and the sight of the retail stores he'd seen from the van windows. The residence staff member did have a number for a cab company and gave it to him. The cab arrived. Tony said, "I told the driver to take me to a cheap motel."

"That's all I knew to do," he continued. "I had not met people when I had a chance at the local AA meetings. I wasn't from Miami, and I didn't open up to the strangers from the neighborhood. It is weird how when you are in recovery at a rehab, you get close to the people in the rehab. My world was the rehab and the other people in rehab. It was co-ed, and that was cool. I really thought I would stay in touch with people I met in rehab. That isn't reality, man."

The cab driver drove north on a wide boulevard toward Fort Lauderdale. "The meter fare was getting pretty high. I didn't want to spend more than a twenty on the cab," Tony said. "I had already made up my mind to get a bottle. When I saw a liquor store a block from a cheap-looking motel, I had the cab stop."

Tony checked in and went right to the liquor store. There, he bought a large bottle of cheap vodka and returned to the motel room, turned on the TV, opened the bottle, and sacked out on the lumpy bed.

I asked, "Why, man? Why'd you do that?"

"That's what I knew how to do." And he rationally explained, "I was a traveling musician and then a truck driver. That's what we do. Stay in cheap places, get drunk and high until the next road trip."

"How long did this go on?" I asked.

"I was there four nights alone, drinking and chain-smoking Camels."

Tony paused for a long moment and looked up at the ceiling, then, with a sigh, said, "My cell phone rang one morning. It was one of the guys I knew from the rehab. Thank God. He said a room was open at the sober house he was staying at and asked if I wanted it. I told him yes. So, I moved in the next morning."

"And...?" I thought there would be more to his story.

"And I started going to AA every day."

"And...?"

"And I have been sober ever since. That was almost eight years ago."

No plan? No ambition? No idea what to do if you are not drinking or drugging? Do you know where you are going to live after rehab? Will you be living alone? Will you be safe there? Can you stay sober there? What people will you live with? What line of work will you be doing or pursuing?

Write the answers to these questions in your exit strategy journal.

Therefore, an exit strategy encourages you to keep a journal of your thoughts and ideas. What you are thinking today is for future reference. There may be a good idea right now that will be forgotten later when you are released and trying to get a perfect life together. Thoughts and ideas are the same as dreams in that they are soon forgotten.

We frequently step into the future without a plan. Plan what you want to do and set realistic goals. But think about what you really want to do. It must be down-to-earth and practical. Discuss it with others. Ask for support if needed. Find people with similar ambitions. If you want to be a pilot, find other pilots.

First, regarding serious life choices and decisions, don't make any too soon. For instance, do not get divorced or married the first month you are out of rehab. Don't move to an unknown or even another city. Make no lifestyle decisions until you are confident and secure about your sobriety.

Change as little as you can as you become accustomed to being out of the treatment center.

You have plenty to change about yourself. You are finding a new you. The people in your life will find a new you, too, if you stay sober in your awareness recovery.

But secondly - and this is a big but! – if any relationship is burdensome, unhealthy, and toxic, then it is better to end it. Say good-bye; it is okay to cry. If something or someone has a negative influence for you emotionally, mentally, or spiritually, letting it go is best.

Shed your past like a snake sheds skin. Get rid of the bad in the past. You will find most of it was encumbering and troublesome anyway. Old resentments and sorrows that you are carrying around will lead you to a bottle of booze or a hit to get high. Baggage does not help you function sober.

Lose your burdensome baggage.

And you know who is harmful to you. It could be a parent, an adult child, a spouse, or a fiancé.

Because there are so many different circumstances, having a coach or counselor who can offer objective opinions and advice will be helpful. Old friends may present a danger. They have their own agenda and vague and unclear motives to keep your relationship alive. They may even resent your recovery. There is too much you have to do now to implement your exit strategy. It will be wasted time and energy trying to guess what is on anyone's mind.

Begin working on your exit strategy by gathering all the literature and notes while in rehab and write everything that is pertinent and valuable to you. You will find that writing insights and thoughts encourages deeper reflection and contemplation and might expose feelings previously unknown. If you are not accustomed to writing, that's okay. Take your time and be patient. Don't worry about spelling and making sense to anyone but yourself. No one is going to read what you are writing. And write everything by hand using pen and paper. This process uses both sides of your brain, right and left. And what you write is more secure on paper than on a computer, tablet, or flash-drive. You will reveal your subconscious thoughts through writing free-form and not editing as you write, as we tend to do on a computer keyboard. This is my best suggestion.

What is written is very personal and sacred.

SACRED

What is sacred to you? Think of something sacred to you. Write down a few things that come to mind. Anything in your world or beyond what you imagine, and that is not to be challenged or disrespected, can be sacred to you. It is something of great personal value that you cherish greatly. The sacred does not have to be something you worship. The sacred must be something you will never harm. A few things that might be sacred are water or air, or your own body, your mind, your family. It might be an object like a guitar, or the Bible, or a location in the wilder-ness, or your home; perhaps your marriage.

Do you know any sacred places? Chaco Canyon in New Mexico is considered by some to be sacred ground. Monument Valley in Arizona and Death Valley in California are included in Sacred Places North America: 108 Destinations by Brad Olsen. Many of the places listed and described are naturally beautiful and awe-inspiring.

There are sacred objects, like crucifixes, chalices, and rosary beads for Catholics. Every religion has its sacred objects.

I have brought up the term "sacred" because in AA Twelve Step recovery, "God" and "Higher Power" are common terms. If you choose to participate in a Twelve Step program after rehab, discovering what is personally sacred is a good way to begin identifying a Higher Power.

Many in recovery struggle with the Higher Power concept and make it too hard for too long.

Holding something to be sacred will help. Why? Because there needs to be something in your life that you refuse to harm and will fight to protect.

It is helpful to have a sense of something greater than you, that you cherish so much that continuing addictive activity would harm what is sacred to you. And you do not want to harm what is now sacred to you. Like your own life. What about your own life? Something sacred could be your body as a temple housing your soul.

Let's revisit your choices. What about your family? Do you have children? Are you married?

Would you consider your marriage sacred? Is your church sacred? Any of these could be seen as sacred. Although you cannot stay sober for someone else, you can stay sober for your own happiness, health, and the relationships you find sacred.

This is part of you living a balanced life.

A BALANCED LIFE

Euripides (480-406 BC), a Greek/Macedonian playwright, is credited with observing, "The best and safest thing is to keep a balance in your life, acknowledge the great powers around us and in us. If you can do that, and live that way, you are really a wise man."

Let's look at what a modern balanced life is and how to achieve it.

1. PHYSICAL

Exercise: Do push-ups, sit-ups, crunches,

jogging or walking, swimming, golf. Frisbee, bowling, and boating will get you off the couch. Lack of physical activity is also one of the main causes of obesity and being overweight.

Rest: Sleep for six to eight hours when you can. Sleep helps the body repair itself. You may personally need more or less, as sleep requirements vary between people. When you feel tired during the day, take a nap or meditate for ten minutes.

Eat: Develop a taste for healthy food. Fruits and raw vegetables, nuts, and seeds are better for you than potato chips and soda water, and they will not promote weight gain. Eating regularly will greatly reduce your craving for and obsession with alcohol and drugs. Food is meant to nourish your body. Real food is nutritious and does not have adverse metabolic effects. Fast food does not meet this requirement, as it harms the body. Junk food is a misnomer, a contradiction, because junk is not food. (Look online and find a food pyramid. There are several competing food pyramids, so pick one or two that you like. Post a copy on your refrigerator as a reminder.)

Relax: Make time to relax periodically during the day. Just lie down and think about what you did before you started relaxing. Think positive thoughts or take up a relaxing hobby. Take your eyes off the computer/tablet monitor at least every hour to relax your eyes. Turn off any noises (TV, radio, including music) and let your ears rest too.

2. MENTAL

Plan: Plan each day ahead of time and set attainable, reasonable, and sensible goals. Keep a to-do list daily. Don't stress out if you don't accomplish everything. Remain flexible and gentle on yourself. Try different approaches to meet goals. Remember, sometimes life just happens. You may not have time for everything. Be as productive as you can. Give each task an hour at least to complete. This way, you will not rush.

Write: Keep a diary or journal. If you have negative thoughts and are angry or sad, let it out on paper. It is a healthy therapy. This gives you greater power. You cannot pretend to be happy all the time. Acknowledge this fact, but don't over-emphasize bad feelings and thoughts. If you feel especially good and enthusiastic, then write that down and relive the good feeling of what is exciting you. Accentuate the positive often.

Discover: Find out about you. Develop your talents. Explore new activities to discover what you like. You might like rock climbing, or you might like knitting; you might like horseback riding, and you might like singing. You never know until you explore. Pursue those activities that agree with your personality, pique your interest or curiosity, and fill you with enthusiasm.

Read: Find a subject you are curious about and read about it. Books, magazines, and newspapers are abundant. There are thousands, if not millions, of fiction writers. Biographies can be fascinating. Try reading classics, such as Shakespeare or Jane Austen. Browse the bookstore or library or Amazon.com; there many subjects. There are thousands of non-fiction writers, too. Books and articles about health, psychology, art, science, auto mechanics, politics, history, philosophy, nutrition and cooking, law, and, of course, substance abuse are plentiful. Then there is the genre of self-help and inspirational books. Authors of this type are Joel Osteen, Stephanie Dowrick, Deepak Chopra, Wayne Dyer, and hundreds more.

Let the book pick you. If you are drawn to it, it was meant to be.

3. SPIRITUAL

Pray: It was not easy for me to pray. I started with the third-step AA prayer suggested on page 63 of the Big Book. Saying this prayer earnestly each morning, I witnessed a difference in the way the day unfolded. It was all good. Then, I began a short prayer before each meal, showing gratitude for my food. Then, I began an evening prayer that gave gratitude for the day I had lived.

Proper prayer requires humility. Honoring the Source of all should always express gratitude for the bounty life gives. No matter how much or small, gratitude should be given by us to the Creator. Effective prayer has a calming effect on your being and promotes overall wellness. Spiritualresearchfoundation.org offers this: "Prayer impacts our spiritual practice at three levels, action, thought and attitude... All actions that are preceded by prayer for spiritual benefit are performed with spiritual emotion; hence, fewer errors are committed... Prayer reduces worry and enhances contemplation."

Prayer is also a good way to express humility and eliminate prideful vanity and delusions of grandeur. Many of us believe in a Creator, a Source of all, yet we balk and shy away from praying. How arrogant are those amongst us who are too prideful to be humble in prayer? Throughout history, greater men and women than you and I have prayed.

Affirmations are another way to have a positive effect on your actions, thoughts, and attitude. If prayer remains not to your liking, then find an affirmation or two. There are books filled with affirmations. Repeat your chosen affirmation several times during the day.

Expressing gratitude is certainly a consciousness-lifting practice. Dr. Margaret McCraw, in her book The Relationship Code, suggests several things anyone can easily be grateful for. For example, she writes, "I am grateful for being alive and knowing that life allows change." And "I am grateful that I am learning to make conscious choices and to release what no longer serves me."

MEDITATE: This practice has numerous physical health benefits and benefits to the physical brain. Master entrepreneur and visionary Russell Simmons had this to say about meditation in an article on Entrepreneur: "Meditation is going to make you happier and more connected to the world. That's what it's done for me, and that makes it the most beautiful gift that I could share with any of you... It's also the most effective tool to help you achieve your goals."

Ringo Starr (of Beatles fame) stated in a 2015 interview that he still meditates every morning at age seventy-five. He began meditating in 1968 when his bandmates, along with Mick Jagger, Donovan, Mia Farrow, and others, studied transcendental meditation with the Maharishi Mahesh Yogi at his ashram in India. Ringo says it is simply a great way to start the day.

Ringo has also taken photographs since the early '60s, as well as being a world-class drummer for sixty years. This is mentioned to encourage you to develop a hobby. There must be more to life than work traffic jams and movies.

Wake up and then meditate? I don't agree that because my eyes are open, I am awake. Wake up first. Have coffee if you like, and breakfast too. Then pause, sit still for ten minutes or twenty -play some gentle instrumental music, or a guided meditation. This way, you will know when ten or twenty minutes have passed.

Allow silence in your life. If you need to wake up thirty minutes before others in the household, do it.

Morning meditation gives your mind-soul-psyche and body the opportunity to become centered, serene, and connected with consciousness before whatever calamity, cacophony, or discord may ensue. Then, it will be met with patience, calm, and peaceful acceptance.

NATURE: Being in the outdoors is good for you.

It grounds you by connecting you with the planet Earth. If you can get to a park, visit there regularly. Go outside, hike, go camping, or fishing. You may find yourself hugging a tree. Frequent time in nature is healthy.

4. SOCIAL WELL-BEING

Do a good deed. Recently, I was walking to the post office and was in a bit of a hurry. I came across an elderly man in a wheelchair. He was stuck on an upward grade in the street. I took a deep breath and decided to slow myself down. The post office would still be there in thirty minutes. I pushed the man in the wheelchair two blocks to his bank.

Be cooperative with other people. Let someone else go first. Listen to people. There is a difference between hearing words and paying attention. Do not resist being helpful every day.

5. FINANCIAL WELL-BEING

Everyone, at one time or another regret when money has been spent carelessly. There is no greater carelessness than drinking, drugging, and gambling, except shopping online, of course - that tops the cake! Considering that this needless waste of financial resources plagues many substance abusers, do this exercise. Pick a number that represents an estimation of approximately how much you spent on your habit each day, then multiply that number by 365. Write the number of that result in your exit strategy journal. Example: 365 multiplied by $40 = $14,600.

Knowledge is power, and educating yourself will help you be independent of others and more confident. Going to school will give you the opportunity to meet new people. And if a new friendship evolves, great, and if they ask you to join them for a beer, just tell them that you don't drink.

A lot of people do not drink.

Study whatever interests you. If you need a new career or want advancement in your current career, take courses. If you want to learn music or art or gardening, find an instructor for lessons. Everything requires learning.

Regaining dignity after years of degrading yourself is challenging. But educating yourself is a great way to raise your self-esteem. The work you do can be performed with confidence and pride, and the way you present yourself in appearance and speech will improve.

Happiness is achieved through accomplish-ment. Get something done well, and you will smile. The accomplishment of learning something new and becoming proficient at it will make you proud and very happy.

What Will You Do?

"If we don't change our direction, we are likely to end up where we are headed."

Ancient Chinese Proverb

GONE ARE THE DAYS OF getting high at dawn and then sleeping till four in the afternoon, then ordering a pizza and ordering more dope, perhaps running to the liquor store while waiting for your orders to be delivered. You are not going to wake up and finish the bottle of vodka from the night before. Those days are gone. You are not going to wake up and roll a joint to start the day. Those days are over.

What will you do?

You will begin with creating a schedule for yourself. Specific tasks and routines for each day of the week will be written down by the hour. The schedule is yours to make. Having a job makes it easier. The objective is to minimize your idle time. If you get bored, you will start remembering your dealer's number or which liquor store has a sale.

These are your instructions. You wrote them, and you want to follow them thoroughly. Start by creating a calendar for Monday through Sunday, with all the hours of the day, and fill in your planned activities, chores, and other responsibilities. If you are fortunate enough to have your own business or employment or are enrolled in classes, many of the hours will be filled easily. That work schedule is one you have already manifested: made reality.

Now, to maintain a sober and balanced lifestyle, your free time must be productive and beneficial and not destructive and wasted.

The mind and body enjoy routine because it reduces stress. Every time you don't know what to do, the confusion causes stress to your brain and body. You may get a headache, and you may feel muscles in your neck tighten. That is why you have made a schedule: to reduce anxiety and tension.

Follow the schedule that you created. It will become habit. Follow your instructions thoroughly.

This is your goal.

GOAL SETTING AND MANIFESTING

Every time that you accomplish a goal, you have manifested a new reality. When your balanced activities become habit, that is a lifestyle newly manifested.

Your end-of-day routine should include an entry in your journal with something of significance that happened, something to be grateful for, and, I strongly suggest, a to-do list. The journal can be as simple as noting one thing of significance that occurred, whether a thought or an experience, or it could be as many details as you can recall and the emotions you felt. A gratitude list can be as simple as one thing that you are grateful for.

First, write down the things you want to do, and then prioritize the things on your list. Give each task an hour. This prevents frustration when you don't have enough time. Especially if driving anywhere is involved. It might even be best to give medical appointments two or three hours.

If you finish any task in less than an hour, do not rush off to the next task. Take that extra ten or fifteen minutes to pause, reflect, and relax. Do an easy meditation. Step outside and breathe the air, or simply sit in silence. Quietly enjoy the feeling of satisfaction that comes with accomplishment.

TIME MANAGEMENT

Paula is a realtor. She wanted or needed one more line of cocaine before making an appointment. Paula did one more line and then rushed out the door and got in her car. She fumbled with her keys while talking on her Bluetooth to confirm the appointment. She intended to show a home to a prospective buyer. The car started, and she backed up hurriedly. There was a car accident ahead of her at the freeway entrance. Paula called her client while stuck in traffic. She arrived late and apologized to the waiting buyer. Paula walked to the front door, nervously talking non-stop, and then, reaching into her handbag, she realized the keys to the house were not with her!

She probably lost that sale.

Time management works hand in hand with the organization. Organization is enhanced with awareness. Slow down. Take a look around. Check twice that you have all that is needed before making your next move. Some people may find your double-checking annoying, but for a while this is good for you. You are at ease knowing. This is, after all, about you.

There is a common phrase: "I will be right back."

There is no such thing as "right back." More likely, this means thirty minutes of driving erratically, with no concern for anyone but rather a single-minded focus on getting more booze or blow. I suggest that you never tell anyone that you will be right back. It makes you an unintentional liar. Increasing awareness of self, time, and environment will make you realize that other than time to pee, there is no such thing as "be right back."

This a good place to rid you of the notion that multitasking exists. Multitasking attempts will make you lie. "I am on it, boss," you hear yourself say on Line 2, while taking notes from another client on the phone and simultaneously completing a travel-expense report, then trying to explain later that 150 was mileage, not the price of lunch. AA's Tradition Five, described in Twelve Steps and Twelve Traditions, states, "...better do one thing supremely well than many badly."

There really is no such thing as "being good" at multitasking. Our attention is always on one thing at a time. And when our attention is divided, then no task receives full attention. Then, it becomes necessary to do that thing again. What we call multitasking is merely a failure to give any one task full attention. Kat McGowan, in her Psychology Today article "Meet the Supertaskers," writes, "The very concept of multitasking is a myth. Our brains don't do two things at once; instead, we rapidly switch between tasks, putting heavy burdens on attention, memory, and focus." She adds, "[A]ttempting to multi-task only ramps up the informational commotion in our minds, creating an interference crisis."

McGowan's article is based on the findings of cognitive psychologist David Strayer of the University of Utah. His research is on the super-tasker. What makes it possible for someone to successfully do more than one thing at a time? What Strayer finds is the elimination of distractions is the essential key.

Try this. Schedule one hour for each item on your to-do list. This will improve your time management and reduce stress during the day.

Having machines has made us believe we are orchestrating tasks in tandem. The dishwasher is washing, the washing machine is washing, the DVD-R is recording Back to the Future (again), and you are sending texts and taking a "selfie" -this is not multitasking. Your mind is not focused on any one thing, and nothing that the machines are doing. If you are, then you suffer from what is commonly called being "scatter-brained," and that's not good.

People often complain they do not have time in one day to do all that needs to be done. Why is that? Because they did not plan the time to do what needs to be done. Make time for what is important. Don't procrastinate - prioritize!

If you find yourself rushing in the morning -wake up earlier. The serenity of quiet time in the morning will become something appreciated, even cherished, after a week or two of practice. Make a to-do list daily. List the things that must get done separately from the tasks you want. Then, devote an hour to each task.

Yes. One hour. If it gets done sooner, then take a break. Pat yourself on the back. Rest or meditate, or contemplate the best way to proceed with the next priority of the day. If the task required you to stand, then sit down, relax, and meditate.

If the task required you to sit, then stand up, stretch your limbs, take a short walk, and relax and breathe deeply.

This is especially important if you work at a computer for hours all day. Your eyes need to look away from the monitor every ten or fifteen minutes. Just gaze into the distance; how far does not matter. The same goes for your hands. Your fingers and wrist need a break more often than every hour. I know these are not easy habits to get used to, but when I developed carpal tunnel syndrome, I learned.

If the task takes longer than you expected (this happens a lot), then that's just the way it is. Accept it. You may need to reprioritize your tasks for the day. It could be that traffic caused a delay of an hour and now you should decide if you should proceed to the dental appointment late or forsake that appointment to pick up the kids on time.

Multi-tasking is a phrase that should be put to sleep. Unfortunately, employers still like to read the phrase on a resume, and so it will remain in our common vernacular.

PATIENCE

Acceptance is very important. Acceptance rejects and shuns resentment. Acquiring patience is difficult, but learning to accept the situation that life presents you is the only mature, positive, and healthful response.

Your impatience leads to frustration. This often leads to anger and venting and reacting in a very immature manner, conjuring and then nurturing a petty resentment that is only in your mind. You have seen this happen in traffic a lot. A driver speeds up to the red light and then honks the car horn the second the light turns green! Immature driver is at large. Is that you?

One of the things that I have come to appreciate is moving at a natural pace. I choose to walk three blocks rather than drive. Travel by car exceeding even thirty miles an hour is unnatural, and airplane travel is completely abnormal to the human condition. Unnatural activity causes stress on our bodies, and our internal organs can become ill due to anxiety, angst, nervousness, and worry. In fact, driving, watching TV, and eating junk food are all unnatural activities, but these are the goings on of our mainstream culture. No wonder we are so often stressed out!

ROUTINE

The mind and the body like routine. Routine is not a rut, unless you do it with negative energy. The routines you set up in your schedule are a big part of your exit strategy. The activities of house chores, employment, business, or leisure must be at the least acceptable to you. It is best to make a routine of washing the dishes soon after eating; that way, the dishes, and pots do not pile up to the point that washing dishes becomes a thirty-minute chore on your schedule. And go ahead and put laundry on your schedule. Laundry can be scheduled in the same time block as taking a walk, exercising, reading, cooking, or meditating. Sleep is vital to good health, sleep, and proper nutrition. Sleep is necessary. Getting sufficient sleep also reduces weight gain and makes obesity considerably less likely.

It is commonly thought that an adult should sleep seven hours each night. When we are agitated and worried about the fate we face, or excited and enthusiastic for the next days' opportunities, sufficient sleep sometimes suffers.

Getting used to sleeping sober can be a challenge. Regular and routine sleep habits must be learned. As with everything else, living sober is a new learning experience, and sleeping sober is no different.

Drinking and doping until comatose may have become the norm.

Does this sound familiar? Smoking and drinking abusively until four o'clock in the morning.

Finally, succumbing to the inevitable reduction of brainwave activity and the body's exhaustion, we passed out. We did wake up eventually, or relied on an alarm clock due to work responsibilities.

There was never time to eat breakfast. We never ate breakfast. A cup of coffee on the way to work or at work would do until lunchtime.

If we did not have a job, then we slept until noon or later and started all over again: drinking and doping. A few of you reading this might relate.

That lifestyle proved detrimental to all aspects of living.

Getting enough sleep is crucial, essential, and vital for wellness. Sleep is the activity that rejuvenates the physical, spiritual, and mental condition of our being. This rejuvenation maximizes our overall health.

What happens when we sleep has everything to do with brainwave frequency, heart rate, breathing, and muscle tension or lack thereof. It has been concluded that there are five stages of sleep in one cycle. We go through the five stages over and over during the course of a night's sleep. If you are a person who dreams, you might be able to relate to these cycles while you sleep. Each cycle lasts about ninety minutes.

Specifically, the stages of sleep are as follows:

Stages 1 and 2 are characterized by theta brainwave activity and constitute light sleep. When you find yourself nodding off in class, you are experiencing light sleep, and if awoken, you will say, "I wasn't asleep."

Stage 1 may last ten seconds or ten minutes.

My stage 1 usually lasts almost ten minutes. This is the transition from wakefulness to sleep. You are partly awake and partly asleep, still aware of your surroundings but slipping into comfortable relaxation. This flows into stage 2, which is characterized by a slowing down of the heart rate, a lessening of muscle tension, and easy breathing.

The theta waves of stages 1 and 2 flows to stages 3 and 4, which are characterized by delta waves. Delta sleep is the deepest sleep we can have. Muscles are completely relaxed.

Heart rate and blood pressure are lowered and body temperature becomes lower. In delta sleep, the body does repairs. Healing, growth, and restoration take place now. In stage 3, less than 50% of the brain waves are at delta frequency, and in stage 4, more than 50% of brain waves are at delta. When a person is talking or walking in their sleep, they are in stage 3 or 4 and very hard to wake up. Have you ever tried to wake someone sleepwalking or -talking? Not easy at all. If the person is awakened, they are very disoriented; they do not know where they are and may not recognize you immediately.

Finally, there is a stage 5, characterized by Rapid Eye Movement (REM) and dreaming.

Here is the way the sleep pattern is understood: stage 1 through 5, then down to theta 4 and 3 and 2, then back up into deep sleep 3 through 5, then repeat. All humans sleep in this cycle. Every human being in the world sleeps like this, every sober human sleeps like this.

Learning to sleep in sobriety can be challenging at first. Here are a few tips that will help. Avoid cigarettes and caffeine in the hours before going to bed. Having a Coca-Cola or a coffee drink and/or a cigarette at midnight is guaranteed to keep you from reaching stage 2 anytime soon.

Eat well at regular intervals daily, but do not eat too soon before bedtime, because digestion requires energy, and expending energy is counter to muscle relaxation and the body's self-restoration and healing functions.

Get off the couch. Be active. Do something each day to make your heart beat fast. Everyone is different. One person may jog two miles while another might walk half a mile; one person may swim two hundred yards while another may have a routine of exercises like pushups, sit-ups, crunches, lunges, and the like. Someone may take up yoga, and someone else may take up kickboxing. I mention this wide range of activities so you can consider one. Regular physical activity will greatly assist in relaxing your body and allowing your brain to slow down and get restful, healthy, deep sleep.

Moving from the couch to the lounge poolside does not constitute an activity.

Our bodies and minds like routine. And we can program and reprogram our routines. Begin a pre-bed habit. Before you retire to sleep, make it a ritual to read for thirty minutes, or brush your teeth and shower, or meditate, or do some floor stretches. Anything done habitually before sleep time will send signals to your brain and body that it is time to go to sleep.

In conjunction with your pre-bed habitual ritual, go to bed and wake up at the same time every day. Even on the days that you don't need to be anywhere soon, get up anyway. You can take a nap later, but your brain and body need discipline and they don't know the difference between Sunday and Wednesday. Treat every day the same with regards to your sleep pattern.

Lastly, make a place that is a sacred space for sleep. Just as you have a gym for working out, a studio for recording music or painting, a place for meditation and a garage for car maintenance, make the place you sleep in perfect for getting good sleep.

In review:

1. **KEEP A TO-DO LIST**

    - Each afternoon or evening, write down the tasks and chores that need to be done the next day.

    - Then write down the things you want to do the next day.

    - Schedule one hour for each item on the list. This is part of learning good time management.

2. **KEEP A DAILY JOURNAL**

    - Where you went

    - Who you spoke with

    - Anything or anyone new you encountered

- Keep a record of any significant dreams

3. KEEP A GRATITUDE LIST

- What you are grateful for (I have a roof over my head; a new car)

- Who you are grateful for (my life partner)

- What or who you would like more of in your life

Write these things down with pen and paper.

This causes a completely different cognitive learning process that promotes memory retention to take place between the brain and the hand.

Do the lists and journals daily until it becomes habit. This can be done in as little as fifteen minutes in the evening.

I encourage you to journal creatively in the morning. When you first wake up from a deep sleep is the time your intuitive thinking is at its peak. This is the time to creatively write your thoughts freely. The time when you first wake is obviously the time that your mind is the most clear and undistracted. Writing in the morning is like having a conversation with yourself. You will write something that comes to mind, reflect on it, and write the next thought. You do not know what will end up on the page. You might remember something from a dream. Write that down. This is therapeutic for you.

Before ending your day, make a to-do list. Do this at the end of each day so you know what to carry over to the next day and what to set as a priority.

I suggest you write what happened during the day each evening. This becomes a diary of events. It is always surprising when I look back through my diary and realize that three things happened in one day, and my memory had spaced them out over a week!

The practice of writing is good for your long-term sobriety, and the to-do list made each evening gives you focus;

when the tasks and chores are completed, you will be pleased to have accomplished and manifested something complete and new. This builds positive self-esteem. Remember that there can be no growth in your comfort zone. Facing challenges and overcoming obstacles builds confidence and good moral character - live to be as near to flawless and impeccable as can be but without stressing about achieving perfection.

Believe in yourself. Do not believe everything you hear. Believe you have the strength to do what is right. Do not believe that you are stuck being a miserable, mean, and miserly person doomed to suffer in mental, emotional, and physical illness due to drinking and drugging for the rest of your life. Every day, life hands you a menu. Today there are only two items on the menu. Oneis Unconditional Love and the other is Chaotic Disarray. What are you going to order today?

Try the unconditional love. It is one of life's specialties.

Smart Choices

"The national taste for alcohol...dated back to the Puritans, whose various modes of purity did not include abstinence. The ship that brought John Winthrop to the Massachusetts Bay Colony in 1630 had more than ten thousand gallons of wine in its hold and carried three times as much beer as water."

LAST CALL: The Rise and Fall of Prohibition, Daniel Okrent

OKRENT FURTHER WRITES, "BY 1763 rum was pouring out of 159 commercial distilleries in New England alone," and, "By 1810 the number of distilleries in the young nation had increased fivefold, to more than fourteen thousand in less than two decades."

Drinking alcoholic beverages was included in daily maintenance by the European colonists, explorers, and traders. It was part of the cultural habit from day one on American shores. Is it any wonder that America celebrates alcohol to this day? Booze has always been part of the social fabric.

In 1632, the children's hospital in Norwich, England, included two gallons of beer in the weekly rations of each child. Certainly, every one of those children suffered dependence on alcohol the remainder of their days.

General George Washington made alcohol a ration for the troops of the Continental Army.

Alcohol maintenance is a dreadful state of being. I know. There's a physical need to drink alcohol even if you don't want to; the delirium tremens demands you make alcohol the master. The opportunity to return to mastery of your brain and body should be welcome and exciting. Are you prepared?

If you do not plan for sober living after rehab, you could end up back in rehab. Don't let that happen. Working with all seriousness on an exit strategy shows your love for you. We all regret choosing anything over love.

Here's a story about not being smart.

Steve buys a new truck. It is a big pick-up. Steve calls up his friend Al and exclaims, "I got a new truck! Do you want to go duck hunting tomorrow?"

"Sure thing," says Al. "What kind of truck you got?" And the two shoot the breeze awhile and make plans.

The next morning before dawn, Steve, Al, and Steve's dog Romper drive out to the lake. The lake is frozen solid. Steve has brought dynamite to blow a hole in the top of the ice, so ducks can land in the water.

They drive the new truck onto the ice of the lake and disembark. "Nice spot. We'll drive to the other side and set up to wait for the ducks, but first..."

And Steve lights the end of a stick of dynamite and throws it almost one hundred yards.

"Nice throw," says Al.

The dog takes off after the stick...of dynamite.

Romper gets to the stick moments after it hits the ice, picks it up in his mouth, and begins wagging his tail and running back with the burning stick.

Al mutters, "Damn!"

Steve exclaims, "Aw, heck no!"

Steve goes to the truck. Al looks bewildered.

Romper is running back fast. Steve takes out his shotgun. Al, bewildered, asks, "What are you going to do?"

"Shoot my dog!" And Steve takes aim at Romper. Fearfully, he fires. Romper keeps coming. Steve pumps his weapon in panic, takes aim, and again fires anxiously. Romper stops, cocks his head to one side, and then starts coming again. Romper is ten yards away when Steve shoots again. Romper skids under the truck with the stick of dynamite still in his mouth. There is no fuse left.

The men survive.

The sudden blast was not surprising, but was immediately startling and scary, to say the least.

Al and Steve were thrown quite a long distance and slid side by side some distance further before the surface ice cracked under the stress, and they became semi-submerged. Steve saw his silver truck sink before swimming and crawling and staggering to shore. There was no trace of Romper.

That evening, Steve called his insurance agent and explained the tragedy. He had been doing business with Sal, his insurance broker, for decades.

They knew each other in college. He thought there would be no problem getting the truck replaced.

Sal said sympathetically, "I wish I could help you, Steve."

A bit surprised, Steve asked almost angrily,

"Why not?"

The agent explained wryly yet dryly, "The truck isn't covered by your insurance policy if you blow it up yourself."

Without an adieu to the agent, Steve hung up.

Silently, Steve sat stunned. He had blown up his own truck. His dog was dead.

His wife called out from another room, "Is everything okay, honey?"

A voice in his head said, "Steve. Calm down. We need a drink."

SMART

In Good Without God, author Greg Epstein describes who SMART (Self-Management and Recovery Training) is for: "any kind of addict who is uncomfortable with or not interested in focusing on the 'higher power' found in Twelve Step programs can turn to a wonderful secular (not religious) alternative, designed by Humanists, called SMART Recovery."

SMART Recovery has local meetings where people can meet face to face. What makes SMART different in one way is that all and any kind of addiction can be addressed. Gambling, sex, and eating disorders, as well as alcohol and drug abuse, are all addictions that SMART meetings are willing to address. And there are online meetings, webinars, and chat rooms.

Here is a comment from a member of SMART:

If you are looking for help with addiction recovery, whether it's addiction to substances or addiction to behaviors, SMART Recovery On-line is a wonderful place to start. Our program is science-based, incorporating scientific best practices in psychology. Here, you will find a supportive online community (message board forums, 24/7 chat, and daily online meetings). We also offer practical tools to help you think your way through what you want for your life and how to go about achieving it. And, like other addiction recovery programs, SMART Recovery Online is free and accessible from home. It may be the only resource you need!

What is SMART Recovery?

SMART Recovery is a non-profit organization. The organization offers addiction recovery support that is founded on scientific research. There local meetings world-wide. The SMART website intro-duces an international recovery community. This includes free self-help support in online meetings.

The SMART Recovery 4-Point Program offers tools and techniques for:

1. Building and maintaining motivation to address addiction related issues

2. Coping with urges

3. Managing thoughts, feelings and behaviors

4. Living a balanced life

What follows was taken from http://blog.smartrecovery.org:

SMART Recovery began (in the mid 1990's) when a group of psychologists, frustrated at what they saw as the limits of twelve-step meetings, de-vised an alternative protocol. It synthesized techniques long used by therapists into four basic points: building and maintaining motivation; coping with urges; managing thoughts, feelings, and behaviors; and living a balanced life.

A SMART Meeting may start like this.

Welcome! My name is Tom. I will be facilitating this SMART Recovery® meeting tonight. SMART is an acronym for Self-Management and Recovery Training. I'm passing around a meeting outline, so you will know what to expect. These meetings will last 90 minutes and are to anyone. You are not required to participate or use your name if you don't wish to. There is no charge for this meeting, but we will gladly accept your donation when we pass the hat later. Our central topic is how to abstain from any type of addictive behavior, including alcohol, drugs, and activities such as gambling. We view recovery as our own responsibility.

We teach self-empowering skills designed to help you: a) build and maintain motivation, b) cope with urges, c) identify and solve the other problems in your life, d) and achieve lifestyle balance to prevent relapse.

Patrick Garnett spent years fighting a losing battle against crystal meth. He went to hun-dreds of twelve-step meetings, sometimes twice a day, but relapse always followed.

Then, about four years ago, an Internet search pointed Garnett toward something different: SMART Recovery, a self-help group whose analytical, science-based methods differ markedly from those of Alcoholics Anonymous and other twelve-step programs.

I went to a meeting, and it was as if the stars aligned for me," said Garnett, 46, who now leads a Chicago meeting himself. "The principles and foundations that SMART is built upon is how I, my partner, and my friends see the world. It just made so much sense to me, and I just felt from the first meeting that this is where I should be.

There are many support groups and alternatives to Twelve Step recovery that stand ready to help people overcome their addiction to substances and behaviors. Each program has merit, and the best outcome occurs when an individual selects a program that best matches their needs and principles or ethics. (Note: some people find that a combination of programs is more helpful to them than a single program.)

For more information, visit: smartrecovery.org/

Below are other support groups for addiction recovery.

CELEBRATE RECOVERY (celebraterecovery.com) describes its program as:

[A] biblical and balanced program that helps us overcome our hurts, hang-ups, and habits. It is based on the actual words of Jesus rather than psychological theory. 25 years ago, Saddleback Church launched Celebrate Recovery with 43 people. It was designed as a program to help those struggling with hurts, habits, and hang-ups by showing them the loving power of Jesus Christ through a recovery process. Celebrate Recovery has helped more than 17000 people at Saddleback, attracting over 70% of its members from outside the church. Eighty-five percent of the people who go through the program stay with the church, and nearly half serve as church volunteers. Celebrate Recovery is now in over 20,000 churches worldwide!

WOMEN FOR SOBRIETY (WFS), a non-profit organization, describes itself as:

Dedicated to helping women overcome alcoholism and other addictions. It is, in fact, the first national self-help program for women alcoholics. Our "New Life" Program helps achieve sobriety and sustain ongoing recovery. WFS has been providing services to women alcoholics since July 1976. The WFS "New Life" Program grew out of one woman's search for sobriety.

WFS self-help groups are found across this coun-try and abroad. Based upon a Thirteen Statement Program of positivity that encourages emotional and spiritual growth, the "New Life" Program has been extremely effective in helping women overcome their addictions and embrace a new positive lifestyle.

This is the first and only self-help program accounting for the special problems women have in recovery, specifically the need for feelings of self-value and self-worth, and the need to expatiate feelings of guilt and humiliation. Their purpose is to help all women with addiction through the discovery of self, gained by sharing experiences, hopes, and encouragement with other women in similar circumstances. The "New Life" Acceptance Program includes thirteen statements to aid those participating in the program, and can be found on their website.

More information is available at womenforsobriety.org

SECULAR ORGANIZATIONS FOR SOBRIETY/SAVE OURSELVES (SOS) takes a self-empowerment approach to recovery, and addresses sobriety (abstinence) as "Priority One, no matter what!" The program credits the individual for achieving and maintaining his/her own sobriety, and respects recovery in any form. There are six suggested guidelines for sobriety, including "Sobriety is our priority" and "We are each responsible for our lives and our sobriety." The others can be found on their website: www.sossobriety.org.

LIFERING (lifering.org) offers sober, secular self-help to abstain from alcohol and non-medically-indicated drugs by "relying on our own power and the support of others." The program operates according to the "3S" Philosophy: 1. Sobriety, 2. Secularity, 3. Self-Help. Meetings are friendly, confidential, non-judgmental gatherings of peers, and the atmosphere is relaxed, practical, and positive. There are meetings throughout the United States and Canada and select other countries. Their description follows:

LifeRing Secular Recovery is an abstinence-based, worldwide network of individuals seeking to live in recovery from addiction to alcohol or to other non-medically indicated drugs. In LifeRing, we offer each other peer-to-peer support in ways that encourage personal growth and continued learning through personal empowerment. Our approach is based on developing, refining, and sharing our own personal strategies for continued abstinence and crafting a rewarding life in recovery. In short, we are sober, secular, and self-directed.

MODERATION MANAGEMENT (MM) offers education, behavioral change techniques, and peer support for problem drinkers seeking to decrease their drinking - whether to moderate levels or to total abstinence. MM offers a variety of behavioral methods for change, guidelines for responsible drinking, and tools to measure progress. The program follows 9 Steps Toward Moderation and Positive Lifestyle Changes, which can be found on their website. See moderation.org for more information.

Some of the programs mentioned here are not as widely available as twelve-step programs (AA, NA, and CA), but they are available to anyone with an Internet connection. Each program offers online services in addition to meetings. Addiction can create huge health and legal problems, and personal relationships suffer. The good news is that there are many pathways to recovery, and many options available, and everyone deserves to find what works best for them.

Who is Rational?

"What's going on here?" asks Moe. Larry says, "We got a flat tire." Curly observes, "It is only flat on one side."

THE THREE STOOGES, American vaudeville and comedy team

THIS CHAPTER WILL INTRODUCE RATIONAL Recovery (RR). Here, there is no God or Higher Power. The acronym NHP (no higher power) is one of the characteristics RR is proud to declare. No meetings, no prayer, and no program of Twelve Steps. And in RR, there is no disease called alcoholism! There is no recovery.

There is only abstinence.

Now, does that get your attention? Does that spark an interest?

A description of an Alcoholics Anonymous (AA) meeting is appropriate here to contrast the spiritual AA and the reasonable and logical program of Rational Recovery (RR). The chapters after this one will discuss AA.

This AA meeting had the group discussion that teetered between the rational and the irrational, the natural and the supernatural. The topic of the meeting was taken from "The Doctor's Opinion" in the AA Big Book.

Jennifer was the chairperson at this noontime meeting. She sat at a desk in front of the assembled members. Nearly eighty chairs were lined up in rows facing the chairperson's desk. There were assorted chairs along the walls and a comfortable couch by the entrance. I saw James, Joseph, and Jerome sitting in a row at the back of the room.

Jesus was pouring a cup of coffee nearby.

A member of the fellowship read the following passage from page xxviii in the Big Book.

Men and women drink essentially because they like the effect produced by alcohol. The sensation is so elusive that, while they admit it is injurious, they cannot, after a time, differentiate the true from the false. To them, their alcoholic life seems a normal one. They are restless, irritable, and discontented, unless they can again experience the sense of ease and comfort which comes at once by taking a few drinks - drinks which they see others taking with impunity.

After describing the cycle of craving, spree, and remorse, the paragraph ends with this sentence: "This is repeated over and over, and unless this person can experience an entire psychic change, there is very little hope of his recovery.

The very next paragraph states, "once a psychic change has occurred, the very same person who seemed doomed, suddenly finds himself easily able to control his desire for alcohol, the only effort necessary being that required to follow a few simple rules".

Jennifer and the attendees thanked Michelle in unison for reading.

One of the interesting phenomena in an AA meeting that begins with a reading from AA literature is that there are many topics available with the reading of only two or three paragraphs.

In the case of this reading, the topic could have been drawn from the first sentence about liking the effect of alcohol, the lack of ability to tell true from false, or even being restless, irritable, and discontented. In this meeting, the topic landed squarely on psychic change.

Michelle asked a member named Jake (another "J" name) if he cared to share his experience on the topic, and he selected psychic change to be the topic. There could have been a variety of topics to choose from, but psychic change is popular in meetings and is a topic that allows discussion of the solution.

Jake began by explaining that he likes psychic change because it deals with what is human. The word "psychic" deals with the human mind. Unlike the term "spiritual experience," which deals with the supernaturalism of spirit. Jake stated clearly that a psychic change means to change one's mind.

"It turns out that it wasn't that I could not do heroin and I could drink or that I could drink and not smoke weed. The fact that smacked me in the face happened in my second AA meeting. I heard these fellas talking, and I started listening. And I realized that I could not do any of it: no drinking, no smoking, no shooting anything. At all! I could not go try anything moderately! Man, I had a real psychic change - clear as a bell ringing. I could not do any of it!"

Jessica took the topic to the spiritual-experience arena when she described the message she heard while in a nebulous state of consciousness due to a drug overdose. She said that a voice very clearly told her, "You can go now if you want. But your son will know that his mom died a junkie." Jessica said that when she came to consciousness, she remembered those words. And she knew then that she'd had a spiritual experience that made her wake up to the fact that she had to quit everything. Jessica said, "I had to admit I would never be able to drink Jack Daniels and snort coke like a lady!"

The members laughed, and Jessica added, "I know you probably don't believe me, but I know that was God who told me that."

The examples given here of people sharing on a topic in a meeting demonstrate how interpretation varies with personal experiences. The fact that "psychic" has to do with the human mind and, therefore is well studied in the world of psychology makes Rational Recovery, a program based on a psychotherapeutic system, reasonable.

RATIONAL-EMOTIVE BEHAVIOR THERAPY (REBT)

Rational Recovery (RR) is grounded in Rational-Emotive Behavior Therapy (REBT).

Both RR and REBT have the trait of being pushy in practice. They both have the objective of helping you "to get it." I like these traits because I, too, intend to push, prod, and poke you long enough for you to develop an exit strategy for yourself that you can and will put into action.

Albert Ellis, Ph.D., devised Rational-Emotive Behavior Therapy in 1955 and introduced it in 1966 with the publication of Rational Living. Dr. Ellis is one of the most prolific twentieth-century psychologists; he is the author of more than seventy books and eight hundred articles. REBT is taught in universities worldwide alongside Gestalt, Cognitive, Narrative, and other systems of psychotherapy. REBT is featured in Theories of Counseling and Psychotherapy: A Case Approach, authored by Nancy L. Murdock.

Unlike AA, whose foundation is in the Christian-based Oxford Group, Rational Recovery is founded in the psychotherapy system developed by Albert Ellis. In his later writings, Ellis was inclined to admit that philosophically, REBT and Tibetan Buddhism did share some common ground. It was 1983 that Ellis published the Journal of Rational-Emotive Therapy, drawing on the 1966 Rational Living publication. Seventeen years passed between these two publications, during which time Ellis practiced his theory in counseling and tightened the case for REBT.

The Albert Ellis Institute website (rebt.org)

states:

REBT is an action-oriented psychotherapy that teaches individuals to identify, challenge, and replace their self-defeating thoughts and attitudes with healthier thinking that will promote emotional well-being and goal achievement. REBT was developed in 1955 by Dr. Albert Ellis. Dr. Ellis has been considered one of the most influential psychotherapists in history. In a survey conducted in 1982 among approximately 800 American clinical and counseling psychologists, Albert Ellis was considered even more influential in the field than Sigmund Freud. Prior to his death in 2007, Psychology Today described him as the "great-est living psychologist."

Greek sage and Stoic philosopher Epictetus is paraphrased by Dr. Ellis in his summary of REBT: "It's never the events that happen that make us disturbed, but our view of them."

The REBT therapist wants the client to learn five things. I want you to learn them.

1. Accept yourself without condition: this is unconditional self-acceptance.

2. Develop tolerance, even high tolerance, for things that you find frustrating; there is not any reason for you to feel bad because you believe something should be different.

3. Accept others just the way they are and without any conditions. This is unconditional acceptance of others.

4. Make a commitment to something outside of your own self: people, things, places, or even ideas.

5. Identify and distinguish your rational beliefs and irrational beliefs (with a coach/counselor if needed), and then take responsibility for your thoughts and actions.

Work at these five things daily.

By writing down your beliefs, and by keeping a daily journal and the weekly gratitude lists that I encourage you to do, you will reveal things of which you were unaware about YOU.

Ellis was a rebel in psychology. His book The Myth of Self-Esteem was published in 2005, two years before his death. This publication asks the question, "Is self-esteem a disease?" Radical that he is, Ellis makes the case that self-esteem is a myth, a fabrication. He sees self-esteem as the greatest disturbance of human emotions ever known. We praise ourselves when we are approved by others and damn ourselves when others disapprove of us.

Ellis says what we need is not self-esteem but rather self-acceptance!

RATIONAL RECOVERY

Rational Recovery (RR) was founded in 1986 by clinical social worker Jack Trimpey.

In 1989, Trimpey published The Small Book: A Revolutionary Alternative for Overcoming Alcohol and Drug Dependence. He published a second book in 1996 titled Rational Recovery - The New Cure for Substance Addiction - The Revolutionary Alternative to Alcoholics Anonymous.

The keyword in RR is abstinence. Abstinence is the practice of refraining from the use of alcohol and any other drug. It also refers to stopping addictive behaviors, such as overeating and gambling.

Trimpey puts forth a way to end alcohol and drug addiction that involves the Big Plan and Addictive Voice Recognition Technique (AVRT). RR has no prayer, no God, no meetings, and no...well, anything that AA suggests is totally rejected and refuted. RR states that to quit abusing chemical substances, one must decide to change his or her mind about using alcohol and drugs, then make a permanent commitment to abstinence, and then resolutely and simply stick with it.

In RR, changing one's mind is within the capability of most every independent individual. The fact that people throughout history have done things or quit doing things because they made up their mind to do so is a fact to be recognized. It is blatantly obvious. People make up their minds to do something and do it. Why not make up one's mind about not using alcohol and drugs? This reasoning pervades the awareness of RR.

Theological or spiritual elements are not central or even important to being rational. RR asserts that abstaining from alcohol and drug abuse is easy when a person remains mindful of the consequences that drinking and drugging brings to their life.

To my understanding, here are the basics of Addictive Voice Recognition Technique (AVRT).

AVRT has you listen to your thoughts, hear your own self think. When a thought occurs that is against your better judgment, identify it and negate it. Recognize it is a negative thought, then negate it: delete it. It is harmful to your well-being. If you allow this negative thought to continue, then you are likely to act on it. The wellness of your being is, foremost, the primary concern, paramount.

So, negate the negative voice in your mind. This voice is your animal: your lower consciousness lusting greedily to be fed. Trimpey calls this animal consciousness the Beast, a lowly dumb part of every human. Your higher consciousness is superior. Your higher-self is stronger than the Beast within. You are the master. You administer discipline. In AVRT, you control your mind. And by controlling your mind you control your emotional responses and actions. You behave in a disciplined, responsible, and independent manner.

Your Beast only wants to survive, but you want more than that. You want to live life healthfully. And you have made up your mind about this. Am I right?

Trimpey's book Rational Recovery: The New Cure for Substance Addiction provides some bullets for your Beast. One bullet is to "clear your mind of everything you 'know' about substance addiction. Focus only on your own behavior and the consequences you experience from drinking or drugging." Another is "Your Addictive Voice is your body talking to you, in thoughts and feelings, telling you to drink or use drugs. It is the sole cause of your substance addiction." And "Recognize that your Beast is ruthless. It cares for nothing you love. It wants only one thing - the pleasure of alcohol or drugs. It will exploit any tragedy, take advantage of any good fortune, to get you to drink or use."

I really like this bullet: Trimpey writes, "Your Beast must use pronouns to get what it wants, and its favorite pronoun is 'I.' Whenever you hear 'I want a drink,' recognize that 'it,' your enemy, wants a drink."

Your response should be "No, I do not want a drink," and wait for it...you will hear the Beast voice try another pronoun by saying, "You want a drink," and when that doesn't work, the Beast will beg "We really need a drink!"

Let it die of thirst.

In RR, with AVRT, you are the boss.

RR emphasizes individual independence. This excerpt from the Small Book states this philosophy clearly: "In RR, you are given the means to reject dependence as a matter of principle and to form a personal philosophy that is by definition conducive to a durable, fulfilling sobriety in which you will independently pursue your own goals."

RR does not dissuade persons of religious conviction from RR. And AVRT is a system that works. Neither does RR persuade or require a person to assume a life philosophy that differs from the one you have. The individual's rights to their own independent mind are respected. There is no suggestion to "come to believe," and there is no supernatural entity (Higher Power) or experienced person (sponsor) on which to be dependent in quitting drinking and drugging.

The dependence demanded of AA members:

Dependence on God, dependence on a sponsor, and dependence on the fellowship meetings, twelve-steps, and service work is criticized and rebuked by RR.

A man meeting a person using RR may well be encouraged to "go ahead" when he or she says they are thinking about drinking that evening.

And "tell us how it goes" might be the response he receives. In another example of RR at work taken from The Small Book, a client in session with a REBT counselor draws this conclusion: "If I loved myself, I'd have a good reason to avoid alcohol because I know what the stuff does to me. If I drank, I'd be harming someone I really cared about - me!"

Me! You!

The revelation is that you (I) are (am) an independent individual, with a fully functioning mind, capable of making good decisions for this life and carrying them out because considerable value is placed on this life. In fact, the value is so great that this life is sacred.

Trimpey admittedly hesitated to use the word sacred, but just as I found, there are some things that are...sacred. There is simply no other word that conveys reverence as well. Here is the excerpt from TSB. If you should have a lapse of judgment and drink or use drugs, you will be acutely aware that you have violated a covenant with yourself that is next to sacred. All right, let's call it sacred. You can say that your life is sacred if nothing else is. Biologically, this makes sense, because we are programmed for survival.

What is Rational?

"The difference between stupidity and genius is that genius has its limits."

ALEXANDRE DUMAS, French writer

RATIONAL RECOVERY ADVISES THAT THERE is no such thing as an alcoholic. RR strongly advises that you never label yourself an alcoholic or an addict.

Do not say this in court to lawyers or judges, to employers or family members, or even therapists.

Don't say you are an alcoholic or an addict expecting some special consideration; you may get special treatment in a way you don't want.

There is reasonable cause for this caution.

The words "alcoholic" and "addict" are, for many people, the descriptions of someone with a handicap. An alcoholic or addict is mentally disturbed, weak-minded, immoral, and not to be trusted, often physically sick and emotionally immature. And these qualities may be true of you, but whether they are or not, you have no control of others' perception. More reason to never admit you have a problem with booze or dope by saying that you are an alcoholic or an addict.

Keep your baggage to yourself. And do not label you.

Improve yourself without telling everyone or anyone what your personal objective for self-improvement or spiritual quest is. That is my advice. People, no matter what respectable moral character they present to the outside world, are inclined to talk about other people.

This someone you told your stuff to turns around talking, and your information is retold to another person unknown to you. And your moment of honesty and vulnerability with this person may be revealed to be harmful later. It happens.

Let me simplify. Here is a for instance. You have a job. You want to leave early one day to meet with your psychologist, and instead of lying and saying you have a dentist appointment, you casually and loosely, with an utter lapse of restraint, tell your colleague, "Yeah, I got to go see my shrink at six, and she's across town."

The next day, you are called into a superior's office, and this authority figure says, "I just wanted to see how you are doing?" Her or his eyes are uncomfortably watching you in an examining manner like a doctor's. And all you think to say is, "Everything's great. But that project concerning the..." And you are interrupted: "Don't you worry about that. That will all work out. I guess I just wanted to say hello. We don't talk often." And then you are dismissed with, "I'll let you get back to work now."

And you walk out of the office wondering what the heck that was about. And you think, "I need a drink." Where'd that come from?

Trimpey writes, "When you decide to quit drinking and using for good, the recovery game is over." He adds that the abstinent life will still be affected by the usual life factors such as nutrition, exercise, recreation, relationships, psychological improvements, and spiritual growth. That's life. But it's life without booze and dope on your mind.

My observation is that spiritual growth is indicated by being a responsible adult: exhibiting maturity in thought and action.

Therefore, Awareness Recovery includes tips and suggests ideas to help you address life issues with a focus on behavior. Your exit strategy will encourage spiritual growth through healthful action because there can be no misdiagnosis in this prescription. All you should do is make up your mind to walk two miles every evening. Then do it, instead of watching television reruns of The Big Bang Theory and Friends, and you will have a spiritual awakening or a psychic change. It does not matter what you call it - a shift of attention - just if you implement positive change through actionable behavior.

Take action. The adage is true: action speaks louder than words. You do the action - say you take up jogging, yoga, skydiving, or learning acupuncture - and a change of consciousness will take place in you. A change in behavior will change the way you think and the way you perceive things.

People in our society usually start drinking and drugging in their early teens. Stunted emotional growth is called arrested development. Arrested development began when you started drinking and drugging at an early age. That's why you and the people you party with cry over spilt milk and crumbled cookies.

By missing out on experiences that would have helped you mature, when you were instead stoned and off in the la-la land of your altered state of mind, you missed a growing moment (maybe many). Already, you have noticed, perhaps, that with only a few weeks or months free of alcohol or drugs, you are reconsidering your viewpoint about this or that. Now you can catch up with the other adults by quitting drinking and drugging, boozing and doping.

RR points out some clear benefits to choose abstinence.

- Abstinence is risk-free. It eliminates many troubles, like problems at work or in relationships. It nearly 100% eliminates the risk of arrests, feeling sick, depression or anxiety, paranoia and irrational fear, and anger.

- The result of abstinent living is always sobriety. And abstinence is easier than moderate drinking.

- Abstinence leads to mature behavior 24/7.

- Being mentally clear becomes preferred. Mental acuity and self-awareness fosters confidence. And you start liking being this way 24/7.

- Once this higher consciousness becomes your standard mode of operating with sharpened senses and enhanced skill level, it is hard to seek or desire immoral depravity, sloth, greedy decadence, and gluttony again.

89

RR perceives and points out a few illusions in Twelve Step recovery. One illusion is that attending meetings where people talk about themselves are necessary to stay sober. And although the AA literature states the only requirement for membership is a desire to stop drinking, this also implies that members and newcomers have not decided to quit.

Another illusion is that chemical dependence, addiction, and substance abuse are interchangeable terms meaning the same thing. Chemical dependency is far from substance abuse. A person under medical or psychiatric care may very well be dependent on a drug. Anything from heart disease, high cholesterol, or bipolar disorder may require a drug prescription to assist someone live a safe and healthy life. Substance abuse, on the other hand, is always someone else's opinion that cannot be proved.

This is easily demonstrated when we observe that some people can drink three or four beers at one sitting and be fine. Meanwhile, someone across the room (minding none of their own business) will suggest to the bartender, "You might want to 'cut them off' from any more beer."

Addiction treatment is another illusion RR notes in that it infers that professional help is needed, but what type of treatment is needed is always unknown. All options are on the table. Because of this, everything is explored in addiction treatment: family counseling, group therapy, support groups, self-help groups, one-on-one counseling, or even medication.

One problem that exists in addiction treatment is that psychological or physical disorders could be occurring simultaneously with the misuse of alcohol and drugs. And these problems are real and not identified because the focus is on substance addiction. This is a dual diagnosis.

Some people continue to use due to other problems that remain undetected until society and family perceive an alcohol or drug problem. Physical, mental, emotional, verbal, and sexual abuses may have occurred or are still present in the person's life. And these cannot be expressed openly. The shame and depression they feel gets drowned. There may be a physical condition of which the pain is being medicated. The cause for the substance use is not addressed with the diagnosis of addiction and addiction treatment.

If you suspect there is a problem after you are abstinent, seek professional counseling. Something that drove you to drink and drug may need to be addressed. The good news is that, sober, you can face reality and deal with it. You cannot go back on your RR Big Plan. You made a commitment to YOU.

The dual-diagnosis is removed when you become sober through permanent abstinence with the Big Plan.

This is an excerpt from the RR (rational.org) website.

What is addiction? Addiction is a voluntary behavior (such as drinking alcohol or using drugs) that persists against your own better judgment. Thus, addiction cannot be "diagnosed" or attributed to you by others, including physicians. It is solely up to you to decide if your drinking threatens or harms others and yourself. You must decide now whether continuing your addictive pleasures is worth the destruction that will likely result. In other words, you are free to choose between drinking and not drinking - between the high life and family life, between right and wrong.

Trimpey asks this question, which, he points out, "probably annoys you": "Why do you drink so much when you know the harm it causes you?"

The answer, as everyone knows, and Trimpey does too, is, "We drink and drug for pleasure."

This makes sense. If you are happy you want to get happier with celebration. If you are sad, you want to forget the problem at hand; it will be a pleasure not to think. If you are in physical pain, it will be pleasurable to become oblivious to the backache, toothache, heartache, or whatever.

The continued search for immediate gratification and pleasure becomes habitual. It is not addiction. It is habit. The habit is to make every moment of every day one of unending pleasure. That delusional thinking is why harm continues to come. Financial and medical health, physical and mental and moral fortitude are diminished, often to the point of failure.

Planning your permanent abstinence is a good way to go. Why not? No meetings, no prayers, and no morality check-ups to keep you sane. Can you do it on your own?

RR GROUPS

The following is taken from the Rational Recovery website (rational.org).

There are no Rational Recovery groups, anywhere! We disbanded the Rational Recovery Self-Help Network during the 1990's because addiction recovery is impossible under the guidance of people who have not recovered themselves. Consequently, there are no Rational Recovery® groups anywhere in the world!

Recovery groups are anti-family, and strive to become your new, surrogate family based upon the beliefs and values of addicted people, which are the opposite of your original family values. Your drinking/using problem will be transformed into chronic, lifetime addiction in one meeting, and you'll take on a new addict identity, drop your last name except for an initial, and take on a new last name, "Imanalcoholic," for example, "Hi, I'm (so-and-so) Imanalcoholic." You'll learn to shift the blame for your addiction onto your family with quack disease theories, codependency non-sense, enablers, bad genes, rotten childhoods, etc.

Therefore, attending a recovery group is like trying to learn how to swim by jumping into a pool full of non-swimmers. They will pull you down every time, and you'll die without learning how to swim. These are just a few thoughts to get your wheels turning in the right direction after many years of being frozen in the moral rust of addiction.

A FEW TERMS, ACCORDING TO RR

Alcoholics Anonymous:

1) A group of formerly addicted people who desire to help others quit drinking or using.

2) A recovery club for people who have not made a personal commitment to lifetime abstinence.

3) Alcoholics Anonymous is an intensely religious, secret organization with a creed that states it is not a religion.

Higher Power: A euphemism for a Supreme

Being, Allah, God Almighty, is described in considerable detail in the Talmud, Koran, and New Testament.

- Issues: In the recovery movement, a euphemism for reality, or for personal problems.

- Rational: The use of intelligence and reason to solve problems, as in, Rational Recovery teaches the skill of planned abstinence.

- Substance abuse: 1) Abnormal, aberrant, or excessive use of alcohol or drugs. 2) Someone else's opinion about an individual's use of certain substances.

- Treatment: 1) A method applied to solve psychological, medical, and other clinical problems. 2) An agreement between a counselor and client that the client will continue to drink or use drugs for an indefinite period, at least until certain for-a-fee, therapeutic exercises are to be performed. 3) Addiction treatment is a historic curiosity of the middle to late twentieth century.

- Bill Wilson was a cofounder of AA. It was while under the influence of the hallucinogen belladonna, administered in a hospital as an aversion therapy, he had a profound beatific (ecstatic) vision he later interpreted as a God-inspired spiritual awakening. He joined a Christian fundamentalist sect called the Oxford Group...he bowed out of that group and formed a nearly identical sect, based on the same ideology... These are Jack Trimpsey's definitions of terms used in widespread and common recovery programs. He opposes the concept of recovery and the disease concept entirely. Once a person chooses permanent abstinence, the game of self-therapeutic recovery, as he says, is over.

If you are interested in Rational Recovery, get the books and read them, or visit the website rational.org and download information from there. Find an REBT counselor, someone familiar with Dr. Albert Ellis, to get you started if you feel it will help.

If you are a thinking person and, value your independence, are self-motivated and goal-oriented, you can live sober by choosing permanent abstinence.

Don't concern yourself with what anyone else thinks. Life is so much more lively, fun, and exciting when not intoxicated. You will be very pleasantly surprised. When you have money to go to dinner or take a vacation instead of two grams of cocaine, you will know what I mean. If the job needs a little extra time spent on a project you can put your mind to the task instead of worrying what time the liquor store closes. When someone asks for your help you can be helpful instead of passed out and incapacitated. When your children ask for your attention, you won't mind showing them love.

Here's a question. Does the warrior fight harder for love of country (self) and family or in hatred for the enemy? The answer is the option with love at stake. The enemy is barely known. You cannot hate the enemy sufficiently to die in battle against the enemy. The motivator for victory is self-preservation, saving family, community, and country because these are your love(s).

Accepting that there are areas of your life that need improvement and that there are characteristics about you that need renewing, remodeling, or replacing is the first step in learning to love yourself. With honest and humble self-love, you can win.

Here is a response from RR's founder, Jack Trimpey, to an inquiry I made via email. Jack replied the same day!

August 18, 2014

I suggest you put aside The Small Book, because it was written before AVRT grew up into the powerfully simple approach it is today. Stick with RR: The New Cure, and then be sure to watch the RR website closely for the new book, Rational Recovery from Any Addiction: AVRT Primer, which will come out in digital format, PDF, and Kindle, very soon, probably in September.

You might also subscribe to the Rational Recovery Discussion Forums, a password protected discussion of AVRT-based recovery where you can look in on others involved with AVRT.

Let me know if you have any questions. Jack Trimpey

Who Is Anonymous?

"Respect your efforts, respect yourself. Self-respect leads to self-discipline. When you have both firmly under your belt, that's real power."

CLINT EASTWOOD, American actor

THERE IS A STORY OF a war general landing his troops on the enemy shore and then burning the ships they arrived in. The war general told his troops that there is no retreat. There is only victory or death. Can you imagine the dissent amongst the warriors at the general's command? They knew then that their leader was crazy. So what? They had to face reality. And fighting to the death was the reality they faced.

Think about it. The situation for you is much the same in recovery. Quit or don't. Win or lose; there is no draw.

An image that exists to this day is that members of AA are daily drinkers who meet to talk about their inability to quit drinking. That could not be further from the truth! AA members are people who have found a solution to stop drinking, and meetings are a way of supporting each other and welcoming new members.

This chapter provides a basic introduction for people who have no knowledge of Alcoholics Anonymous (AA) and its program to recover from substance abuse: specifically, alcohol.

AA is a wonderful organization. I enjoy the camaraderie that comes with regular attendance to the meetings. No organization has been more successful in helping people live sober lives. I attended my first meeting in 1989, and to my surprise, there was my lawyer. I was in a month-long outpatient program at that time. The lawyer was attending to the defense of my Driving While Intoxicated (DWI) charge.

AA is great. It helps many but some do not care for its spiritual foundation. Here, I will give history and basic principles of the founding and what the program asks of its members.

Why is the word anonymous used? That's because it was a secret back in the beginning days of AA. The men who formed AA had been heavily drinking and abusing, financially succeeding and failing, and suffering indignation and addiction during the years that alcohol was illegal in America. No doubt, they knew the bootleggers, the speakeasies, the politicians, and the profiteers of illegal booze during the 1920s - the roaring twenties.

Everyone wanted to remain anonymous in the 1930s and '40s about anything related to alcoholism. To be an alcoholic was to be scorned.

People were admitted to institutions for the insane when alcohol made them crazy. To be an alcoholic was to be a deplorable drunkard: unworthy of respect and not to be trusted. An alcoholic was of low moral character, weak of mind, and spiritually sick; surely a sinner!

The anonymity of members is intended to place Principles (of moral character) before Personality.

Times have changed.

When AA was formed, the country had just ended an era of prohibition of alcohol in 1933. For the twelve years prior, beginning in 1920, alcohol was manufactured, distributed, and sold illegally. It was like cocaine is today. This ban on booze created bootleggers and speakeasy cafes that were "underground," and "good" people did not break the law. Alcoholics did!

The founder of Alcoholics Anonymous had his first drink of alcohol in 1917 and his last in 1936. Prohibition of alcohol in the USA began in 1918.

And so, Bill Wilson drank himself to ruin during the years that alcohol was illegal. This was the same period in which Sam Walgreen expanded his pharmacy from one store to a nationwide retail outlet by fulfilling doctor prescriptions for alcohol as medicine.

And so, soon after booze was legal again, the men who formed AA had obviously been drinking illegally during the prohibition era to have developed such severe life problems from alcohol abuse. For these reasons, anonymity was emphasized amongst the founding members.

There is no way to discuss sober living and recovery without discussing Alcoholics Anonymous (AA). This organization has become the go-to program for the recovery industry worldwide. AA created the first Twelve Step program for recovery from alcohol. The history below will explain the dates. Since then, many other organizations have adopted and adapted these Twelve Steps to address other dysfunctions.

If you have something sacred, religious ideology, or a strong spiritual foundation, then the AA Twelve Step programs will be a breeze. Atheists, agnostics, and people of a polytheistic faith may find themselves facing a struggle. A loving God or Higher Power is significant to the AA program.

AA HISTORY

Before Alcoholics Anonymous, there was the Oxford Group, and before that, the Temperance Movement. The Oxford Group was founded in 1931 by Dr. Franklin Nathaniel Daniel Buchman. America was still under the federal law of Prohibition, making the manufacturing, distribution, and sale of alcohol illegal. Dr. Franklin Buchman was an American missionary and Lutheran minister of Swiss descent. Before the Oxford Group, he had founded the New Century Christian Fellowship. He was aware of the politics of the century-old Temperance Movement.

1826 was the year the American Temperance Society was formed. It benefited largely because the American population had a renewed interest in religion and morality. Twelve years after its beginnings, the society claimed more than 1,500,000 members. There were, by 1839, more than a dozen temperance journals were being published in the country.

Buchman had a conversion experience in 1908. It was a conversion to heal sinners. In those days, sin was thought to be a disease. Being an alcoholic was a sin. It would be decades before alcoholism would be perceived as a disease.

The Oxford Group's philosophy took on a "fire and brimstone" approach to sermonizing. The national Temperance movement had built great political strength at the turn of the century and became so mighty that U.S. presidential candidates had to cater to them for popular votes.

The Christian message of the Oxford Group held that all people are sinners, but all sinners can be changed. Confession is a prerequisite to change, and the change can directly give access to God. Miracles through God are possible.

This Christian group had "five Cs," and these were the practices of Confidence, Confession, Conviction, Conversion, and Continuance.

Also, they had the Four Absolutes that set a standard for morality: Absolute-Honesty, Absolute-Purity, Absolute-Unselfishness, and Absolute-Love.

Understanding the Christian foundation of AA can explain why many non-Christians balk when introduced to Alcoholics Anonymous. The Christian-based Oxford Group laid the foundation for AA. And to this day there is prayer at every Twelve Step meeting.

People with substance abuse in their lives generally reject, rebuke, refute, and refuse religion. This attitude has not changed since the day the Puritans landed in New England with more than 10,000 gallons of wine aboard ship.

Drinkers and druggies are skeptical of religion's merit in earthly life. The hypocrisy amongst religions becomes so obvious that it is offensive and obnoxious to many drinkers and druggies. Nothing has changed in this regard for hundreds, even thousands, of years. How many times have religious leaders, from evangelists to priests, been found guilty of committing or being complicit in sexual misconduct? The church's greed for financial abundance was first blatantly evident in the Pope's Vatican rule, and even today, America's television Christian ministries giving sermons to hundreds of thousands of believers in arenas exhibit considerable magnificence of wealth, opulence in the name of charity, and Jesus. Church activity can be viewed as disconcerting. And Bill Wilson was no different in his poor opinion of church folk and religious institutions.

Prohibition ended in 1933.

Bill Wilson's entire drinking life from 1917 to 1936 took place during years that paralleled the enforcement of the Volstead Act of October 28, 1919, and the Prohibition Era from January 1920 to 1933.

Wilson stopped two years after prohibition was repealed by Congress with the twenty-first amendment.

In November 1935, when AA founder Bill Wilson was still a steady drunkard drinking gin, an old friend came to visit. His visiting friend was sober.

Bill was highly skeptical of religious faith and its followers. He writes in Bill's Story that his old friend, now sober, looked him straight in the eye when asked about his sober mind and said, "I've got religion."

Wilson writes, "I was aghast. So that was it - last summer an alcoholic crackpot; now, I suspect, a little cracked about religion...the old boy was on fire all right. But bless his heart, let him rant! Besides, my gin would last longer than his preaching."

Bill's Story in the AA Big Book goes on to describe, in no uncertain terms, Wilson's firsthand conversion to his newborn belief in God. He writes, "Thus I was convinced that God is concerned with us humans... At long last I saw, I felt, I believed. Scales of pride and prejudice fell from my eyes. A new world view came into view." And he also tells us, "I humbly offered myself to God, as I then understood Him, to do with me as He would."

Two things in this passage are revealed that are fundamental to AA today. The third step of the Twelve Steps has its beginnings in this paragraph of Bill's Story, which states, "over to the care of God as we understood Him."

Bill Wilson saw an exit strategy through prayer to God.

It is important to remember that the Oxford Group and Alcoholics Anonymous are Christian-based fellowships. When AA offers members to have a God of their own understanding they are still (most all the time) referring to a Christian God.

The reason that Wilson's third step gives freedom of interpretation of God, concerning a God of one's own understanding, is so critical is amongst Christian denominations, the worship of Jesus as God or not as God but the Son of God or the Messiah is not a point of cohesive agreement. Christians debate the meaning of God, who God is, and how God works even amongst themselves!

Some AA members integrate a religious practice with their Twelve Step program.

It remains that modern AA is known to be the most effective treatment for recovery from alcoholism. Finding a spiritual life in sobriety is important to recovery in AA. As generous as it is that members can have any God, the text still uses the word "God" and capitalizes references to "Him."

Christianity is the foundation for AA.

Because of the popularity of Twelve Step programs of recovery, the Christian origins are obscured so that addicts of all kinds, Buddhists and Jews and non-believers in God, can participate in Twelve Step recovery.

It is the AA Third Tradition that tells the story of how the first atheist member could join AA after much discussion amongst its founding Christian-faith fellowship. The question surely had to be, "How can this man give his life to a God in prayer if he does not have a God?" Still, after much debate, the atheist was allowed membership, and he did get sober.

In AA's beginning, three men were critical to the formation and development of the fellowship Alcoholics Anonymous. They are Dr. William Silkworth, William Griffith

Wilson, and Dr. Robert Smith. Today, Wilson and Smith are known casually as Bill W. and Dr. Bob and deemed the cofounders of AA.

It was Dr. William Silkworth who treated Bill Wilson on one of many hospitalizations Bill W. would endure. Dr. Silkworth had his theories about alcoholic abuse and addiction and, having formed a conclusion, he explained to Bill W. that alcoholism was an illness: a disease.

This was a radical departure from the commonly held belief in Christian America that alcoholism was a moral failure, a sin, and that insanity was the devil's doing.

Silkworth determined that alcoholism was not a failure of morality or willpower. His letter is included in the AA Big Book and is titled "The Doctor's Opinion."

I suggest you read it if you have any interest in AA's Twelve Step program of recovery.

Dr. Silkworth believed that alcoholics suffered from a psychological obsession, which combined with an allergy that made compulsive and continuous drinking inevitable.

To break the cycle of abuse, a person had to completely abstain from alcohol use. This is permanent abstinence. Silkworth's idea, when coupled with a sudden spiritual "hot flash" (which Bill W. experienced while under the influence of the belladonna cure, a drug treatment that had hallucinogenic properties), resulted in a spiritual conversion to God for Bill W.

Bill Wilson writes, "God comes to most men gradually, but His impact on me was sudden and profound."

Bill W. launched with God's fervor a mission to share this concept of alcoholism as a disease and the idea that complete abstinence and prayer could hold the disease in remission. He zealously went about to alcoholics, many in hospitals, sharing this message.

The story of AA's beginnings goes on, with Bill Wilson soon finding Dr. Bob. And together, they set out to save other alcoholics from the suffering, insanity, and death that are the results of prolonged alcohol abuse. The history of Alcoholics Anonymous is well documented in other books and films, and many books offer interpretations of the Twelve Step program and instructions for how to work it.

It is clear that America's Prohibition Era produced a great many alcoholics, both men and women. The wealthy lived it up large, but the poor were sold wood alcohol, grain alcohol, and even anti-freeze. These poisons would get watered down and doctored with something like caramel to change and enhance the taste. A great many illnesses and deaths were suffered.

It is also a fact that in the years between 1920 to 1933, men made millions in the business of alcohol. Walgreens and other pharmacies sold alcohol as "medicine" with a doctor's prescription. Doctors found writing the prescription easy enough for a person suffering night sweats and delirium tremens (DTs). Saloons had been abolished, but "speakeasies" abounded in every major urban city. From San Francisco, Denver, St Louis, the Southern states, and all New England to Chicago, Detroit, Philadelphia, and, of course, New York City, people did openly drink alcohol. It is reported that three speakeasy establishments were located on the same block as one New York City police precinct headquarters.

The way we drink today is greatly influenced by what occurred in America a century ago. Men and women began, for the first time, to gather together for the sole purpose of drinking alcohol and flirting and gossiping. That's when the term "to party" got invented. Before that people did not gather for drink; there was always food. Not long after Prohibition was law, young men of the cities got in the habit of carrying a flask of gin or other liquor always. It got so that by 1923, a young woman could not be bothered with a young man who did not have a flask!

Nowadays, most all people seeking to recover from alcoholism or drug addiction have heard of the Twelve Steps. Many seeking to recover have read the Twelve Steps. But relatively few have worked the Twelve Steps. Working the steps is why members encourage sponsorship.

First, there were six basic steps. The straightforward nature of these six steps is admirable. Note that the word God is not used until the last step. The word God moves into the third step when the steps become twelve.

1. We admitted that we were licked, that we were powerless over alcohol.

2. We made a moral inventory of our defects or sins.

3. We confessed or shared our shortcomings with another person in confidence.

4. We made restitution to all those we had harmed by our drinking.

5. We tried to help other alcoholics, with no thought of reward in money or prestige.

6. We prayed to whatever God we thought there was for power to practice these precepts.

The story is that Bill W. decided that these steps should be made simpler. He was inspired by the number twelve because there are twelve apostles in the New Testament. Here are the Twelve Steps with their guiding principle.

THE TWELVE STEPS AND PRINCIPLES

1. We admitted we were powerless over alcohol - that our lives had become unmanageable.

2. Honesty

3. Came to believe that a power greater than ourselves could restore us to sanity. Hope

4. To the care of God made a decision to turn our will and our lives over as we understood Him. Faith

5. Made a searching and fearless moral inventory of ourselves. Courage

6. Admitted to God, to ourselves, and to another human

being the exact nature of our wrongs. Integrity

7. Were entirely ready to have God remove all these defects of character. Willingness

8. Humbly asked Him to remove our shortcomings. Humility

9. Made a list of all persons we had harmed, and became willing to make amends to them all. Reflection

10. Made direct amends to such people whenever possible, except when to do so would injure them or others. Forgiveness

11. Continued to take personal inventory and, when we were wrong, promptly admitted it.

12. Acceptance

13. Sought through prayer and meditation to improve our conscious contact with God as we understood Him, praying only for knowledge of His will for us and the power to carry that out. Spirituality

14. Having had a spiritual awakening as the result of these steps, we tried to carry this message to alcoholics, and practice these principles in all our affairs. Service

Steps 1, 2, and 3 should not be that difficult if you can acknowledge the mistakes you made under the influence of your substance of choice, that you acted crazy a lot, and have lost any sense of God. These steps are the opportunity to admit you desire to be sane again and able to evaluate the effects of your actions, and will ask for supernatural guidance from a God of your understanding to be your first support in this concern of your life. You will attempt to have faith in the unseen, just as you do with oxygen and electricity, to supply your needs.

Step 4 begins the action part of the AA recovery program. It should not take long after completing the fourth-step inventory to complete 5, 6, and 7. The inventory is simply a written list of traits your character/personality possesses or, especially, lacks. The lacking traits are flaws or defects of moral, ethical character that prevent and deter you from completeness: wholeness.

Step 8 was started in Step 4 with the names of people you have resentment toward. Step 8 only says to make a list. Step 9 is when you attempt to repair the damage done. Making amends is too often interpreted as making a verbal apology. In some instances, this is sufficient, but to wholly repair the damage done, making amends means to make it right: repay the loan, repair the vehicle you wrecked, and stuff like that.

Step 10, 11, and 12 are the maintenance steps for daily living. Step 10 suggests that you apologize immediately if you offend or harm someone, and that at the end of the day, you review your behavior, thinking, and emotional responses to see where there was an error or where you could have done better. Step 11 is plain and there is little room for misunderstanding - daily prayer and meditation. If nothing else, read the AA Big Book's pages 83 through 88 each morning or evening. Carefully read for full comprehension and pause for reflection; your intentional, thorough contemplation of these principles will result in an inner connection with the higher self, Source, and God.

Step 12 is an entire chapter, Working with Others, that discusses this important aspect of Twelve Step recovery. Within the fellowship, there is an action called a "twelfth-step call." This means to go to someone, be it their home or hospital or anywhere, and spend time talking with a person suffering from alcohol abuse. This person may be sick from alcohol poisoning or some other condition that has handicapped their ability to function. The twelfth step specifically refers to helping other alcoholics and sponsorship, but more casually, it extends to the community and society. Be useful, helpful, and of service to others.

Newcomers will also be encouraged to complete ninety meetings in ninety days. This is a good idea. If you can, then do it. Being immersed in the company of sober people and people with the same agenda will keep you focused. You will become familiar with the program's fellowship aspect. In addition, socializing will get you out of your head. And it is medically known that it takes about three months for the body to reprogram and recondition itself to a new regimen: habit, diet, or exercise.

Give yourself three months. After this period, your body will have adapted. You are past the point of painful physical withdrawal symptoms and, hopefully, mental obsession. You have gotten comfortable with being uncomfortable at times. There is no desire to self-medicate. The understanding has come to you that there is no need to add anything to life. This is what it means to live life on life's terms.

What Is Sponsor?

DON STOPPED TO SAY HELLO to Jason at the mattress store Jason managed. Ten minutes later, he said hello to Jody as they walked into the AA meeting together. Jim and John were already there and seated. Jake was making coffee. Jay sat by the back door, making conversation with Jill. Jay was Don's sponsor. Don knew the old guy Jay was a dirty old man and could not resist getting close to a woman, but he knew how to stay sober.

Tattoo Jack had something to share during the meeting about seeing a flower in the desert and feeling God's presence. After the meeting Don spoke with Jerry for a while, and he told Jerry about the winter solstice full moon having a rainbow circle around it.

Then, Don stopped in with Jerome after the meeting. Jerome sold refurbished desktop computers seven days a week. He and Jerome had clicked right away. They talked about open-carry firearms being legal in Texas as of January 1 and software upgrades.

Don was walking home when he thought, "Jesus, I have a lot of friends with 'J' names."

Checking his voice messages, he found Darryl, Dick, David, and Dan had called. They were all on the same bowling team, called the Daring Ds.

Five of the guys with "J" names were on another bowling team. That was how they'd chosen teams. Twice a month during the winter months, they would all go bowling after a meeting. This had gone on for three years. All guys until Janet joined the Rolling Js and Debbie joined the Daring Ds.

Despite meeting at a bowling alley where beer and liquor was served, not one member on either team had chosen to drink. It was their way of making the statement that fun did not require booze.

Getting a sponsor is strongly suggested, encour-aged, and advised. Some members will insist that a newcomer get a sponsor immediately. Some do not. It really is your choice. When you feel comfortable, seek a sponsor. Intuitively, you will find someone you are attracted to. Sometimes AA members will approach you and ask if you need a sponsor. This may be their intuition at work.

A sponsor is beneficial in helping to understand what Twelve Step work is and what is to be done in each step. You can also thoroughly read the basic text of the Big Book, find detailed explanation and instruction in the book Twelve Steps and Twelve Traditions, ask questions of members before and after meetings, and get along just fine and be happily sober. Sponsorship, in my opinion, is your independent, individual choice.

A few things are true about seeking a sponsor and building that relationship.

The sponsor's purpose is to provide instruction on how to work the Twelve Steps and to help prevent you from drinking. Not necessarily to stop you, but to talk you down like a negotiator with the police would talk a "jumper" down from a high-rise building. These two purposes (step work and preventing relapse) are only fulfilled if you ask your sponsor questions.

Meet with your sponsor regularly in person, and touch bases with telephone calls, text, or email to build the relationship. Remember that the sponsor with years of sobriety has a life outside of AA. And they are likely sponsoring others. Don't ask your sponsor for money, food, housing, or to baby-sit your children or feed your cat. Stay on the topic of recovery, and a healthy relationship, even friendship, can occur.

Don't worry if, after a few meetings, you ask someone to sponsor you, and they say no. Sometimes the person has other people they are sponsoring. And sometimes, they do not think you are ready for their sponsorship. Don't worry if the relationship with your sponsor does not work. Get another one. Some sponsors will be proactive and very demanding and will rigorously drive a newcomer through the steps. Some sponsors will wait for you to approach them with questions or call them when you have a craving to drink or drug. Some will call to "check-in" with you. Never be offended. Whatever their style of sponsorship is reflects their personality. Getting a new personality or changing to "please" another, or even being well-liked, is not your main concern. Don't worry about a thing. Everything is going to be all right. Just make up your mind to not use/abuse alcohol and drugs. Everything becomes clearer with abstinence.

No one's feelings will be hurt if you change sponsors if it is handled in a mature manner. Another fact about sponsor relationships is that as a newcomer, the person you choose may be more helpful if they have a few years of sobriety instead of decades of sobriety. Why? The reason is that those AA members with decades of sobriety have often forgotten what it is like being a newcomer. The AA member with only two or three years of sobriety will likely be much more enthusiastic and communicative.Sponsorship has changed from the early days of AA.

Membership to attend the meetings in the 1940s required a current AA member introduce a new member. This was to assure that the new man was acceptable; the existing member would vouch for the new man's character and social standing.

Only proper alcoholics could attain membership in early AA days. Only through an introduction by a proper current member could a new man join. The member making the introduction became the new man's sponsor. If the new man exhibited poor behavior and subsequently failed to quit drinking, it was a reflection on the sponsor.

AA was quite exclusive in its formative months and, perhaps, years. The men who formed this fellowship, despite having once drunk with the privilege of country clubs and golf clubs, had also spent years in impoverished, derelict, irresponsible drunkenness.

Once a man became a member in those days, he went to work on the steps immediately. There was none of what we see today. These days are different. A newcomer may regularly attend meetings and, after nine months, still be searching (lackadaisically) for a Higher Power! And, incomprehensibly, reciting prayers at the beginning and the closing of meetings!

Those founding members would find the way we operate today hard to believe.

We Americans have become too fat and lazy in the past fifty years. We are soft. Our predecessors, having come through a depression and a world war, and being familiar with country living where work chores were daily and nothing came easy, could not take anything for granted. Today, our work ethic and the way we apply ourselves to tasks or schedules, even to save a life, is, in general, quite frankly, slothful.

America and its citizens are in despair, disrepair. Today, more than ever, because women have joined the ranks of alcohol and drug abusers, a majority of Americans wake up with a drug and go to sleep with a drug. We want something, whether cocaine or coffee, to pick us up and give us energy, and then bourbon and Valium to relax or render us unconscious, ends the day. Legally, the prescriptions are many for battling sleep insomnia.

We all know of Ambien, but there is also Doxepin (Silenor), Temazepam (Restoril), Eszopiclone (Lunesta), Zolpidem (Edluar), Zaleplon (Sonata), and Triazolam (Halcion).

Could it be that if we were not jacked up on coffee and cocaine, we would have less trouble sleeping?

And another change in American society is the relief from

racial segregation. That form of societal structure was law until the late 1960s. Neither Chinese, African-Americans, nor Mexicans drank, ate, or spent leisure or recreational time with white folk of any economic status. Even the Irish and Italians were not fully integrated for many decades into white society. Every aspect of life in America throughout the 1940s, '50s, and '60s was segregated by race and religion. European Jews were always viewed with skepticism in America. It was always clear in America what being white was, and white was always right. English, Dutch, Scandinavians, Russians, and Germans were white, and then the French were borderline acceptable, but the southern Europeans of Spain, Portugal, Italy, Greece, Armenia, Turkey, and the Slavic peoples weren't white enough until many years later.

There is no reason to expect AA's founding members to behave any different than the society at large. These founding gentlemen already had the social stigma of being alcoholics: helpless, weak-minded, morally corrupt drunkards. Why would they risk their reputation further by inviting a Chinese, a black, or a Mexican man into their homes? In those days, a non-white could not enter a white neighborhood without white police or other intimidation. That is a fact. That is just the way it was. Can you imagine it?

The fact is that in the beginning, AA was a secret group of white men in the United States. And they wanted to remain anonymous. They did not want the community at large, men of business, courts of law, and others, to know they were heavy drinkers striving to become sober men. These men relied on a Christian God and Christian principles. To say AA was and is a sect of Christianity is not an error.

Bill W. and Dr. Bob, the two men who formed AA, may have been leaning to agnosticism at points in their lives, but that changed dramatically. When they began seeking to tell other men about their ideology of alcoholism as a disease and not a moral shortcoming or sin, they dealt the hand of God.

When the third and then the fourth man joined, they also were white men with Christian values. Not just anyone could join AA. Twelve Steps and Twelve Traditions characterizes this in Tradition Three, page 140: "So, beggars, tramps, asylum inmates, prisoners, queers, plain crackpots, and fallen women were definitely out. Yes sir, we'd cater only to pure and respectable alcoholics!"

White women were even excluded and told to form their own groups!

If these men had not changed their ways and attitudes, then today, atheists, Buddhists, ex-convicts, all women, homosexuals, African-Americans, Mexicans, and anyone who was not a white male would still not be considered for membership.

Bill W. himself wrote that AA sought to help proper alcoholics. He would later laugh at himself about that opinion. On page 140 of Twelve Steps and Twelve Traditions is written, "[T]here was nothing funny about the situation then. We were grim because we felt our lives and homes were threatened, and that was no laughing matter."

Thank goodness, this secret society mentality changed. Today, AA is all-inclusive. Anyone can join. "You are an A.A. member if you say so," page 139 of Twelve Steps and Twelve Traditions states.

Today, AA and other Twelve Step groups are racially and sexually integrated. There are still men's and women's segregated meetings if you care to find them. And, quite naturally, there are meetings predominately attended by one ethnic group or another. These are by mere chance of the community in which they are formed. There are no longer intentionally racially segregated AA meetings.

So, feel free to go to any meeting. The more meetings you go to, the better, because you will become familiar with the diversity amongst groups, and you will be socializing with sober people. One meeting may be boring, and another may bring you into the light of God's grace.

The following is an excerpt from Bill's Story. "I was to sit quietly when in doubt, asking only for direction and strength to meet my problems as He would have me. Never was I to pray for myself, except as my requests bore on my usefulness to others."

Bill's Story describes Bill Wilson's awakening to a spiritual way of living. This was very new to him. Read this chapter to understand the spiritual conversion of this AA founder.

"There Is A Solution" is the Big Book's second chapter, and it contains the following passages written from the first-person point of view "we," as the group had formed and was coming together in the writing and editing of the Big Book.

The great fact is just this...we have had deep and effective spiritual experiences which have revolutionized our whole attitude toward life, toward our fellows and toward God's Universe. The central fact of our lives today is the absolute certainty that our Creator has entered into our hearts and lives in a way which is indeed miraculous.

The Big Book chapter "How It Works" says on page 62, "God was going to be our Director. He is the Principal; we are His agents. He is the Father, and we are His children." As I made clear earlier, if you have a belief in a patriarchal God, no matter what that God is, then AA will be easy.

There is a less male-dominated rendition of Alcoholics Anonymous. This book is for women, gays, trans-genders, and others who prefer God is not a He.

A Simple Program: A Contemporary Translation of the Book Alcoholics Anonymous, written by AA member "J," is the Big Book without male gender bias.

Here are two reviews.

By Caroline McKinnon, writer/blogger, July 26,

2011:

This book was written in 1996, and I did not hear about it until 2011 when an "old timer" at a meeting slipped me a note about it. I came into the program in 1984, and while I was grateful for the new perspective on life after I managed to keep the plug in the jug with the help of AA, I nevertheless found myself struggling with the male dominated terminology and presumption of alcoholics being male throughout much of the text. It didn't feel like "one drunk talking to another" so much as one guy talking to another, so I found it a challenge to fully relate to the truth that I, as a woman, who still had a family and a business and a home, was also an alcoholic. I am very grateful to "J" for adjusting the gender aspects of the language in such a way that any newcomer, male or female, can truly experience the "one with all" spirit that AA is supposed to embrace.

By Ocean "Ocean" (Houston, TX, USA):

This book explains what it means to be an Alco-holic. Being an Alcoholic is as much an attitude towards yourself and life, as a craving for alcohol. For the many who are at the bottom looking for answers, or to the skeptic who isn't sure whether they are an Alcoholic, this book offers clear an-swers to a confusing problem.

I bought this book one day after experiencing a wonderful hangover, and then it sat on my bookshelf unread for years. I read the book while drinking a glass of wine. As I turned the pages, I realized more and more the exact measure of how much I had lost control of my life, and the capacity I possessed for lying to myself.

Spend 12 dollars for a 12 pack and have fun tonight, or spend 12 dollars on this book and learn what it takes to have fun for the rest of your life... real fun.

AA is a spiritual program. AA rejects being called a religion. It is a spiritual program based on spiritual principles. These principles are those in the Twelve Steps.

The following is from "Working with Others" in the Big Book, page 98: "Burn the idea into the consciousness of every man that he can get well regardless of anyone. The only condition is that he trusts in God and clean house."

The social interaction and the friends that you make can be a real pleasure. People laughing in sobriety, like the survivors of an earthquake, telling stories of escaping near disaster is common. After years of either isolating or only socializing with other people that are stoned or drunk, you may find sober conversations refreshing. The trick is to go to different meetings and at different times until you find a group that you are comfortable with. Age, substance abuse (alcohol vs. narcotics), economics, gender, sexual preference, and ethnicity may or may not be important. Don't be afraid. Meetings are safer than a lot of places you have been.

If you are lucky, you will find a Twelve Step meeting group that works in their sharing to offer solutions to life. Often, it comes down to reliance on a higher power. You will be happy to know perhaps that amongst the fellowship there are those who believe that the kingdom of heaven is within and the higher power is there as well. It is known as your higher consciousness.

It only works if you work it. And like the Nike slogan, "Just do it!"

One of the elements of AA that is agreeable to me is the practice of prayer. I find praying daily and even intermittently throughout one's waking hours wise. To keep one's Mind-Soul-Psyche (MSP) focused on the goodness within the supernatural invisible God in which one has faith keeps one's own consciousness vibrating at a higher level. This way, you live in higher God consciousness. And it is in this way that you successfully live honestly and harmlessly. Love and tolerance and kindness and humility are what you exhibit when the practice of prayer is common.

Praying nowadays does return my MSP to memories of Catholic childhood days. There is nothing wrong with those days in my memory. Piety was learned. The virtues of goodness and faithfulness were well worth learning. These qualities are assets to me in sober life. The lessons of honesty - being truthful and kind and generous and giving of love - were learned at a young, innocent age. That means before puberty.

116

That innocent child I was is the one I hold sacred today. That is my real inner MSP. The one I was born to be on earth.

No Elevator

"Step with care and great tact, and remember that Life's a Great Balancing Act."

DR. SEUSS, author

AA PREAMBLE

Alcoholics Anonymous is a fellowship of men and women who share their experience, strength, and hope with each other that they may solve their common problem and help others to recover from alcoholism. The only requirement for membership is a desire to stop drinking. There are no dues or fees for AA membership; we are self-supporting through our own contributions. AA is not allied with any sect, denomination, politics, organization, or institution; does not wish to engage in any controversy; neither endorses nor opposes any causes. Our primary purpose is to stay sober and help other alcoholics to achieve sobriety.

This preamble has been read at the beginning of every AA meeting I have ever attended. The AA logo is a triangle representing unity, service, and recovery: fellowship meetings, helping other alcoholics, and Twelve Step work.

The program of AA is built on the foundation of Twelve Steps. AA is the originator of Twelve Step programs because the founders of AA wrote the Twelve Steps. The Twelve Steps are grounded in moral principles. When these principles are applied to daily living, they promote and support sobriety. These principles are honesty, hope, faith, courage, integrity, willingness, humility, reflection, forgiveness, acceptance, spirituality, and service.

It is instantly clear that anyone living a life based on these moral principles will have a hard time getting drunk or stoned, wasted or high. The twelve qualities of moral character are desirable to have and lead to an elevated consciousness.

This may anger some modern-day AA members, but that doesn't and shouldn't matter to you.

118

The fact is that it does not require half a year or more to complete the work of the Twelve Steps. The first three steps are simple admission that you have a problem, and your life is a mess, and that you want to be sane again and you are willing to let God handle your life. An unmanageable life is apparent when your mortgage/rent are in arrears; the utilities of electric, gas, and water are on notice of being interrupted; you have become homeless; you are seemingly unemployable, or your pride prevents you from working for less than you dream you deserve; your personal and intimate relationships are only troublesome and angry, or there are no friends any longer. These are some of the clear signs of a life in disarray, unmanageable.

The first three steps could be done, by anyone ready to quit drinking/drugging, in a few hours over coffee with another member (sponsor). Don't get stuck on Step 3: "Made a decision to turn our will and our lives over as we understood Him."

What you understand about God will be different for most every other person on earth. Personally, my understanding is a God that has no gender. My Higher Power is not male (him) or female (her).

That is because my God does not need to reproduce.

That's just my understanding.

Steps 4, 5, and 6 can be done by that evening's mealtime or at least within a few days, if it is kept simple. By simple I emphasize that Step 4 need only pertain to current resentments, hatred, and perceived obstacles or struggles. Dredging up ten-or twenty-year-old resentments is not constructive.

I did that once and became so overwhelmed I bought a bottle of booze after three days.

Step 6 is where we willfully and consciously confess we are ready to be rid of the shortcomings and weaknesses revealed in Step 4. This means that you will yourself to end the thinking and doing the actions that you found abhorrent about yourself.

And then Step 7 is where you humble yourself through prayer and ask the God of your understanding to assist you, aid you, and guide you daily to be free. A realistic relationship with and positive perspective of yourself has been achieved by working the first seven steps. It has been humbling to admit that your ways in the past were filled with error and failure.

More self-reflection takes place in Step 8.

Truthfully admitting you have done harm to others and contemplating the manner of that harm and damage done is not easy. Now, to make a list of people you have harmed may take some time. Write the first few names that come to mind. Parents, perhaps siblings or other relatives, and any friends or employers, employees, or co-workers gives you an idea of what you want to consider. Don't forget any intimate relationships, past or present.

Step 9 suggests that amends be made, not simply apologies. Amends means to repair the damage done: make things right.

Saying, "I am sorry I wrecked your car," is not making amends. Paying for the repairs is. When the harm is not tangible and material, it is much harder to mend, to repair emotional and psychological wounds, but an attempt must be made. This frees you from the conscious and subconscious turmoil your soul suffers.

Take a ceramic plate and throw it onto a concrete floor. Did it break? Yes. Now, say you are sorry to the plate. Is the plate repaired? This how hard it is to repair yourself. It takes time to piece it together with glue to wholeness.

Contact people in person. Tell them that you want to make things right. Ask them what will repair the damage. Do this during the week ahead, and Step 9 is done. If you owe someone money, set a date to repay them. If you washed their white shirt with new blue jeans and now the shirt is sky blue, get that person a new white shirt.

There are people on this list that you can make amends with immediately (within a week or month). Then there are those people that you no longer have a way of reaching and cannot make amends with. And lastly, there are those persons that you harmed but to whom making amends would cause more harm than good. The easiest example of this is a former lover or ex-spouse who has entered another relationship or marriage, and their new relationship does not need your intrusion.

Now, begin practicing Steps 10, 11, and 12 in your daily life: every day.

There is another approach to working the steps that some may call heresy.

Do Steps 1, 2, and 3, and learn to practice 10, 11, and 12 at once. The first three prepare you for the new life, and the last three maintain the new life daily.

Do the inventory as suggested in Step 4. Share what you found resentful to you, as suggested in Step 5. Once you come to understand the basis of your resentment(s) and your role (or part), then your own less-than-stellar moral value asks God to remove these faults. This means to make the necessary changes in your beliefs, attitudes, and way of life. Correct yourself. You will be able to think clearly about any resentment you may have. Step 7 concerns itself with humility. Ask God to help you correct the moral failings found within. This is a very significant moral value essential to building desirable character.

Rectifying the past is not an emotionally easy thing to do, so give it another month or two. List people you have harmed, as suggested in Step 8. Then, as the months pass, you will be sober enough at six months to approach someone to make amends as is suggested in Step 9.

Just keep it simple. If you find you missed someone or something in Steps 4 and 8 later, then do those steps again. It's okay to remember stuff after a few months sober and make corrections. The important thing is that you begin practicing the maintenance steps of 10, 11, and 12 as soon as possible.

There is nothing sadder than a member attending weekly meetings for years and telling the group, "I don't know what my Higher Power/God is." And yet they will pray with the group at the end of the meeting!

The saying amongst AA members is, "It works if you work it." The work is thoroughly following instructions. Clear directions are provided. Doing the step work, reading the Big Book, attending meetings, and not picking up the first drink will allow a person to live a sober life quite happily.

AA literature refers to changing one's mind as a spiritual experience, a spiritual awakening, or a psychic change. These terms become topics of endless discussion in meetings. The point is that in recovery, a person must change their mind about using alcohol and drugs. The decision to stop using requires a change of consciousness and a new awareness of life. You must decide that alcohol and drugs have no place in your life.

How will you change your consciousness? You started when you decided that daily drinking, smoking, tooting, or shooting was no longer a way of life that you wanted. You assessed your life and found it no longer functioning well and no longer manageable. You saw that your life was out of control. The only thing that matters is that your life was not acceptable to you.

This is very important. Your high life brought you down and must not be acceptable to you any longer. You will not stay sober for anyone else. You should get sober for you. That's the only way it works. You must passionately desire this lifestyle change.

If you are sick and tired of being sick and tired, out of your mind and out of cash, then you have a chance to change your mind: have a psychic change, a spiritual experience, and get sober.

If you choose AA, then you will begin a spiritual program. There is prayer at the meetings and it is recommended that prayer and meditation become part of your daily life. Step 11 suggests daily prayer and meditation. I recommend making this a habit immediately because it will help clear your mind and make it easier to accept the challenges of all the other steps. Step 12 suggests being of service to others. Begin helping others right away. This will make honesty and humility easier when you work the other steps.

Steps 4 and 5 and then 8 and 9 are the challenges most people struggle with because pride must be humbled. You must be honest.

Four additional books that support the Twelve Step program of recovery are helpful. These are Twelve Steps and Twelve Traditions, Living Sober, As Bill Sees It, and Daily Reflections. All can be accessed online at aa.org and are available in book form at most AA meeting places and bookstores.

There are various types of AA meetings.

Beginner meetings are open to anyone. These meetings are also known as Newcomer meetings. People are encouraged to attend these meetings to learn what AA is about and how sober living is a good choice. One of the things about AA that is attractive is its inclusiveness. Relax when you go to meetings. The people attending are just people. Some are happy and sober.

Newcomers are treated differently in different meetings. Some meetings do not allow newcomers to speak. I have been to those types of meetings. I was told to ask questions after the meeting. So, it varies from city to city, region to region.

Members with long periods of sobriety may or may not be warm and welcoming. Remember that people attending AA meetings are just ordinary people in most respects and have their own troubles. In some places, open arms and generosity is the atmosphere, and in others, "sit down, shut up, and listen" may be the established attitude. "Take the cotton out of your ears and put it in your mouth" is a common old-timer's saying. Don't be daunted. This is your sobriety.

Make new friends when you can and become comfortable with the recovery program of Alcoholics Anonymous. The people you meet at the meetings have experience; most will be helpful in some way.

Open meetings are another type of meeting.

Here, anyone is welcome, whether they are alcoholic or not. This is likely to be the first type of meeting a person in new recovery will attend. Open meetings are the most common type of meetings in most communities. Open meetings allow people with short and long sobriety, newcomers and family members, friends, spouses, and children to learn about AA recovery.

Closed discussion meetings permit only alcoholics to attend.

Step meetings are held so that members learn what each step involves. For example, Step 8 suggests that a member write down a list of names of people he or she has harmed. Step 9 suggests that amends be made to that harmed person.

Not an apology, but amends. Amends means to make right the injury done. If you owe someone a thousand dollars, making amends means to repay the thousand dollars. Saying "I am sorry" does not make amends.

Big Book Study meetings are helpful. Reading the Alcoholics Anonymous Big Book can be a challenge. There are no wasted words in this book. Read for comprehension. Every paragraph contains useful information. Use a dictionary. When I read the third step, I needed to use a dictionary to get the synonym "worry" for the word "care" to help me understand the step.

Speaker meetings can be very inspirational.

The member speaking usually has many years of sobriety. The life stories will include the past behavior under the influence and how living life sober has been beneficial. One speaker meeting I went to featured a deaf woman using sign language. She told the story of using sign language at karaoke bars to get drinks by "signing" the lyrics to the song. The audience loved her. Go figure.

There are inter-group meetings, and regional, statewide, and national conventions and conferences. There are even international conventions.

Reading and studying the AA Big Book is essential. But some people get by with just a sponsor and the book Living Sober.

The Big Book's basic text describes the program.

But the English it uses is so old-fashioned that some people have difficulty. Read it with a dictionary. Many words used in the 1930s are not in common use today.

The book Living Sober is helpful. This little book contains very reasonable and practical answers to common problems people have when adjusting to sober life.

The "cult" stigma surrounding AA still exists in our society. If you feel it is no one else's business (and is not) about your attendance of AA meetings, then tell them it is none of their business, or "Hey! I joined a book club!"

Use the Steps

"The journey of a thousand miles begins with one step."

LAO TZU, Chinese philosopher

ASIDE FROM THE INDIVIDUAL WORDS, there are word phrases that need clarity in AA. Three phrases that people struggle with and many never fully understand are "psychic change," "spiritual experience," and "spiritual awakening."

A psychic change means simply to change one's mind. Psychic comes from the word "psyche." Psyche is the totality of the human mind, both conscious and unconscious. It is the mind.

Psychology is the scientific or objective study of the psyche: the mind.

When the Big Book states that a psychic change is necessary to stop drinking, it only means that a person has changed their mind about drinking or drugging. They have come to believe that getting high has no place in their life.

Spiritual awakening is a separate matter. Step 12 states that spiritual awakening comes because of working the Twelve Steps.

Spiritual awakening means that the mind has awakened to that spirit that is within us and that represents God's presence in life. And so, the person has become God-conscious.

This is a new state of consciousness.

The eleventh step suggests daily prayer and meditation. You are not working the program of recovery as prescribed by AA without doing these two practices. No one can help but have a spiritual awakening eventually if they are praying and meditating earnestly every day. These two activities always result in contact with the Great Spirit of the Universe: God.

It is wise not to allow yourself to be confused by other members in their interpretation of these key phrases: psychic change and spiritual awakening. Their previous experience, education, and personal history are unknown to you.

Keep it simple.

It really is simple. If you have an experience you feel is spiritual, that is great. If not, no big deal.

You stayed sober another day. No one knows what, when, how, or why a spiritual experience occurs. It is personal.

Working Steps 1, 2, and 3 do not require action. They only require honesty, hope, and faith. Step 3 has a prayer associated with it:

God, I offer myself to Thee - to build with me and to do with me as Thou wilt. Relieve me of the bondage of self, that I may better do Thy will. Take away my difficulties, that victory over them may bare witness to those I would help of Thy Power, Thy Love, and Thy Way of life. May I do Thy will always!

When I began saying this prayer, I did notice a difference in the way my day went. Things seemed to go smoother. My luck seemed better. There is no way to know if the day would have gone just as smoothly without the prayer. So, all I can say is, it doesn't hurt to pray.

Prayer and meditation is painless.

Some steps offer promises of what life will bring with the completion of that step. Completing Step 5 will offer the following promises to the person recovering in AA. They are not presented as listed promises as I have written them here, but the words have not been changed. These promises appear in paragraph form on page 75 of the AA Big Book.

- We are delighted

- We can look the world in the eye

- We can be alone at perfect peace and ease

- Our fears fall from us

- We begin to feel the nearness of our creator

- We begin to have a spiritual experience

- We feel the drink problem has disappeared

- We feel we are walking hand in hand with the Spirit of the Universe

These promises are the result of completing Steps 4 and 5. You will hear the term "character defects." This is, unfortunately too often the focus. When you do a personal inventory, look at the good things about yourself as well as the things you think can be improved.

The fourth step can be a real pain in the ass.

It usually results in a member recalling events in their life that they would rather leave forgotten. Newcomers work the inventory as though they are constipated, struggling to get every little pinch of it out. Don't make it that hard.

Here is my best advice. When doing a fourth step, do not go back to childhood. Deal only with your immediate resentments and injuries and the weaknesses and strengths of character you possess today. Unless there is a horrible trauma like sexual molestation, rape, suicide, or a death that has had a significant influence on your life, don't concern yourself with old stuff. Keep it simple.

If you hate your boss, write that down. The fact that you hated your third-grade teacher is insignificant today, right now.

Step 5 scares many newcomers because all the stuff they wrote down in Step 4 is now to be shared with someone. Those little pieces you struggled to push out in Step 4 are not anything anyone else human and the loving God Almighty of your understanding have not seen before floating in a bowl of water.

Many do this Step 5 with their sponsor, but this is not absolutely required. A clergy member or a counselor will do. The main objective in completing Step 5 is to gain integrity, humility, and freedom.

Having the courage to face up to what failures or tragedies are in the past, taking ownership of the good and the bad within you, telling someone and admitting wrongs, and then accepting their response and criticism is a freeing experience.

A new outlook on life often comes after doing this step.

The Step 9 promises appear on pages 83 and 84 of the Big Book.

The eighth and ninth steps reinforce the spiritual principles of reflection and forgiveness.

Step 8 suggests making a list of all persons harmed and Step 9 suggests that the member make direct amends to those persons harmed. Again, these are not comfortable steps to work through. But the rewards are stated clearly in the ninth step promises:

If we are painstaking about this phase of our development, we will be amazed before we are half way through. We are going to know a new freedom and a new happiness. We will not regret the past nor wish to shut the door on it. We will comprehend the word serenity, and we will know peace. No matter how far down the scale we have gone, we will see how our experience can benefit others. That feeling of uselessness and self-pity will disappear. We will lose interest in selfish things and gain interest in our fellows. Self-seeking will slip away. Our whole attitude and outlook upon life will change. Fear of people and of economic insecurity will leave us. We will intuitively know how to handle situations that used to baffle us. We will suddenly realize that God is doing for us what we could not do for ourselves.

Are these extravagant promises? We think not. They are being fulfilled among us- sometimes quickly, sometimes slowly. They will always materialize if we work for them.

The first nine steps provide instruction for conscious living.

Working these steps sober and truthfully will produce positive results.

The book Understanding the Twelve Steps by Terence T. Gorski explains and summarizes the step work. He writes, "As a result of steps one through seven, you have fixed yourself on the inside. Through steps eight and nine, you have fixed what you can on the outside. Now that your lives are back in working order, step ten tells you to watch yourself carefully. When you do something that is harmful to your recovery, fix it immediately."

Step 10 resonates with some of the theories presented later in this book. This passage on page 84 of the Big Book reads, "We have entered the world of the Spirit." We have come to communicate with the Source that is God, which was always within us, but now we are connected to that which is the all.

Step 11 is the daily spiritual action required.

Daily prayer and meditation is the way an AA member maintains a healthy and strong spiritual condition. It took many years for me to grasp the spiritual life of AA, but I did. And I am grateful that I did because it taught me how to live consciously, be aware of what I am thinking and doing, and grateful. I can deal with everything life throws my way with mental clarity and good moral judgment.

AA members admit the Twelve Steps are emotionally challenging. But to recover, the alcoholic must face their fears, and fearing their emotions (fearing their selves) will likely result in a relapse. Not feeling emotions is what drinking and drugging was intended to do. Keeping emotions squashed is why people drink and drug abusively. By the time an AA member is working on Step 11, fear of self is gone, or should be.

The twelfth step involves working with other alcoholics or addicts. Nothing helps keep an alcoholic sober more than working with suffering alcoholics. Service will get you out of yourself. This is healthy. Newcomers are encouraged to get out of the old isolation habits.

Attend ninety meetings in ninety days, and while at the meetings, volunteer to take out trash, make coffee, sweep floors, arrange chairs, and, in general, be of help.

Dr. W.W. Bauer is quoted in the Big Book, 3rd edition, on page 572, as saying, "[T]he alcoholic overcomes his excessive concentration upon himself. Learning to depend upon a higher power and absorb himself in his work with other alcoholics, he remains sober day by day. The days add up into weeks, the weeks into months and years."

The twelfth step states that because of working these steps, a spiritual awakening will have occurred. It really does work, and the promises come true - if the steps are worked. AA will not keep you sober if you do not follow the instructions.

"Working With Others" is an entire chapter in the Big Book. This is essential reading, as it will prevent mistakes from happening when you do attempt to help other alcoholics. People that are using drugs and alcohol are sick people. If your sobriety is frail, you are not likely to be very helpful.

Twelfth-step work is spiritually rewarding.

Helping others always makes a person feel good; just be sure you are ready and willing to help.

Pages 152 to 153 of the Big Book say, "Life will mean something at last," and, "Then you will know what it means to give of yourself that others may survive and rediscover life. You will learn the full meaning of love thy neighbor as thyself."

There is no shame in asking for help.

In Twelve Step meetings, you will hear people share their experiences, strength, and hope, what it was like and what life is like now. Some of this will be helpful and insightful. You will gain awareness about some aspect of your own circumstances.

Your perspective will change about a lot of things when you are sober. After thirty days, it will feel wonderful, and ninety days will be better.

Being able to be reliable and responsible will feel good. You will develop a sense of direction, and the fellowship will give you a sense of belonging. You will not be clueless and without direction.

Yesterday, I sat alone on a bench on a busy city street and observed people. For me, it was motivating because it reminded me of the vast numbers of the population that are busy, busy, busy but directionless, rudderless. Living a sober life in fellowship with AA will give life meaning.

Keep an open mind in meetings, and when you are comfortable, share something to let people know you. Even if you are uncomfortable, go ahead and speak up. Nothing you say is likely to be shocking. Most AA members have seen and known plenty of insanity. By sharing your troubles, you will have a cathartic experience; cleaning up bottled up emotions has to happen somewhere at some time. Getting stuff out really is freeing.

Here is something I heard in an AA meeting.

When a man was checking into a motel the front desk clerk asked, "Can I have someone help you with your luggage?" And the hotel guest replied, "No. I am traveling light."

That's the way you want to be: traveling light in life.

Now you have an overview of what working the Twelve Steps is about.

If you are ready to get started with a Twelve Step program, don't talk about, and don't make excuses.

Just do it. There are meetings everywhere.

And the next time you are in a social situation, and someone asks if you want a drink or a hit, tell them, "No thanks. I have had enough!"

Three words of great significance found in AA literature are "thorough," "rigorous," and "trudge."

We do not use these three words often today. Here is what they mean.

- Thorough means comprehensive, detailed, and systematic. When is the last time you were thorough about anything?

- Rigorous means severe, difficult, and demanding. When is the last time you were rigorous about any task? Most likely, if anything was too demanding, it did not get done. Am I right?

- Trudge means to walk a particular path or distance, with slow and weary steps: a long, exhausting walk. It implies that a burden is being carried. When carrying a load or hauling heavy stuff, we slow down. If we quit we do not reach our goal. What was your last triumphant accomplishment?

These three words - thorough - rigorous - trudge are worth remembering. You may want to remember them because you will want to apply these characteristics to your future efforts in life, and especially when considering your goals. Anything worthwhile achieving in life requires these elements be applied. You must be demanding, relentless, and systematic; even when the load seems too heavy to bare, you must push through to get to the other side: to reach your goal.

What will you pursue with this much effort?

What will you strive for regardless of how strenuous the effort required? Your mind is searching right now, asking you, What? What is it?

The clue is that whatever your goal - you must be passionate about it.

The goal must be one that you can attain by yourself. Do not look for handouts; no one can get you sober! Clarity of thought will come with sober time. In the framework of reality, you will soon be making realistic goals.

Being an astronaut is not a realistic goal. But there are careers in aerospace. Being a sports superstar is probably unlikely, but there is employment in sporting enterprises. The chance to be a supermodel may have passed you by, but making other people look and feel beautiful and glamorous pays very well.

Your goal will be something you can do on your own.

To further your education, seek grants, scholarships, and very small loans. Find out what your passion is and pursue it with passion. If you are not passionate about a goal, your desire will be weak, and your efforts will be minimal. And success will not arrive.

Happiness is achieved with accomplishment.

Are you ready to be happy? Then, set pragmatic goals that you have a burning desire to achieve. The media is filled with stories of persons who come from poverty to wealth. These individuals are living proof that anything can be done in life. If we live in a free society and we keep an open and drug free mind, we have access to unlimited personal power.

Procrastination and laziness was your foe.

Psychologist and philosopher William James wrote in 1886, "Nothing is so (as) fatiguing as the eternal hanging on of an uncompleted task." Isn't that the truth? Week after week passes, and they turn into months and often into years, and you still have not completed something you have told everyone you would do. Always with an excuse about money or time, but all time and money has been spent getting high. The term "pipe dream" is so very appropriate, isn't it?

Now, those foes have been challenged. Your inner strength is becoming more powerful. You are taking the steps to a new life. Continue to build upon your recent experience in rehab. "Creating wealth is never about money; it's about creating freedom," is the philosophy and mindset of Mr.

Kenneth Brown, inspirational speaker, business coach, author, and CEO at Ken Brown International, who in 2014 was financially worth millions.

Here is the opening paragraph of his online LinkedIn profile.

Everyone has a story to tell. Few, however, prove to be as profound and inspirational as that of Mr. Kenneth Brown. He had every excuse to choose a life of failure. At the age of 13 and 14, Ken's parents brought their first child into the world; by 17 and 18, they were mother and father to five children. Despite poverty and a trail of 10 evictions, Ken's parents still emphasized the importance of education and a strong work ethic.

Everyone has a story to tell. That is so true. Mr. Brown and many others have life stories of success. Brown had every excuse to fail, but he chose not to go that road. You can choose a successful life, too.

Awareness Recovery has a few words that will be emphasized throughout. They will be helpful to keep in mind.

One of the words is "sacred." Determine what is sacred to you. Cherish what is sacred and how your sobriety does damage to your relationship to what is sacred in your life. Is it your family? Is your relationship with God sacred? Is your community sacred? Only you can determine what is sacred, and you will not let drunkenness hurt that.

Contemplate what is sacred to you and there your God will be revealed personally.

Another word is "focus." Having clarity of mind will allow you to focus your attention on a task until it is completed.

The third word is "now." This is what time it is. The more awareness you give to the present moment the less the illusions will confuse your thoughts and actions. Yesterday is long gone and only a memory. If mistakes were made, then NOW is when to act to correct the mistake. Tomorrow is a hopeful fantasy, and NOW is the time to plan and schedule events. Stay in the NOW as much as you can, each minute of the hour, each hour of the day. Things will work much better by correcting your past, working in the present, and building a successful and happy future.

As true as water is wet, inner peace and happiness come through accomplishment of purposeful goals, which in time manifest the reality desired.

Solitude Is Not Isolation

"Neither shall they say, Lo here! or, lo there! For behold, the kingdom of God is within you."

KING JAMES BIBLE, LUKE 17:21

THAT WHICH IS NAMED GOD resides within the realm of the human consciousness. God exists in belief. If you do not believe in God, then God does not exist for you. If you believe, then God exists within you. The source is free. God gives you choice. You choose your beliefs and thereby create your reality. It is your consciousness that defines the Universe for you.

Strengthening intuitive consciousness is the objective: the gold we mine. It requires time alone to get the work done. Every miner wants to stake his own claim. You don't want someone else controlling your thoughts and emotions: your consciousness. Stake now your claim to your mind.

When you drive or walk down a street with a tablet or smart phone and earplugs, now your eyes and ears are grossly oblivious to what is coming up ahead of you. I see this behavior all the time. That's an analogy for life under the influence. Drunk or stoned, you can't see clearly what is coming up, and you have forgotten what you just passed and left behind. And you are largely oblivious to the present moment.

This is your life. And you might be spending much of it under the influence of others and subjects that have nothing to do with you. Movies, television court and game shows, college and professional sports, gossip, and rumors of the rich and famous have nothing to do with you. Such topics should be relegated to the category in our mind labeled nonsense. These are entertainments for us, but are not worthy of much attention afterward. Not until I am in the grocery store check-out line do I become distracted by the nonsense of Charlie Sheen's promiscuously sick sex life, Miranda Lambert's smile, Britain's royal family, or flat abs.

Remember to block this junk out of your mind.

You are beginning to live your life anew now.

To live a good life, you will have to learn to love yourself. To love yourself, you have to get to know yourself. To get to know yourself, you have to spend time without the TV, the computer, and the other electronic devices. Twitter and Facebook are not mirrors to your soul.

Albert Einstein said, "Solitude is painful when one is young, but delightful when one is more mature."

Learning about you, loving you, and relying on your intuition are noble objectives. How is this done? Incorporate one or two of these ideas or actions daily, and then include the others until they are daily habitual components of your life and mindset. Self-seeking pleasure need be gone, as well as self-pity. Honesty, open-mindedness, and willingness (as AA suggests) are the characteristics to be treasured.

Developing your intuition requires that you be creative, meditate frequently, listen to your body's yearnings, practice spontaneity and open mindedness, be less opinionated and judgmental, practice being present in the now, get regular exercise, get outdoors, journal, pay attention to your dreams, rest and relax, and eat healthily.

Open a dictionary. Look up the words mind, soul, and psyche. You will find they are synonymous. They refer to the same nebulous being that is you!

Being true that the mind, the soul, and the psyche (MSP) are synonymous, meaning the same in English, then it follows that there exists no divide, separation of, or difference between spiritual growth and mental growth.

Growth of either, spirit or mind, being that they are one, requires knowledge be accessed and acquired, accumulated and retained.

The education of the mind comes in an enormous array of approaches.

Learning comes to all beings first through the senses. Observation, touch, taste, smell, and sound are primary. These faculties inform us well of the outer world in which we live. Awareness of the outer world happens when we are awake, meaning conscious.

Somehow all the things we learn get retained and can be recalled. We choose to call this memory. Memory is a miracle. How does that happen? You tell me, and we will both know. Some psychiatrists, perhaps teamed with neurologists and biologists, I would presume, have researched the science of the mind, written, theorized, and proven a plausible, even popular, concept explaining the miracle of memory.

I am merely in awe of the miracle. And as fascinating as memory and the retention of information is, allowing learning and then knowledge of our outer reality, there is this other thing.

We think. Think of that. Thinking is marvelous when you think about it. What a wonder! It is a phenomenon, don't you think? How does that happen? Again, if you tell me, then we will both know. The same team of scientists, perhaps?

Clearly, by now you understand why my emphasis in Awareness Recovery is on the mind.

The functional mind is really all there is that keeps us creatures of any type (mammal, reptile, bird, and bug) from being lumps of matter wandering and bumping or whatever we would be doing, functioning in a pattern of perpetual cycles of generation and regeneration, birth and life and death. When the mind stops functioning then all the stumbling, wandering, and bumping occurs. That is what we call mindless. Which is a euphemism for insane. And the stumbling, wandering, and bumping is what we do when we are intoxicated by mind-altering drugs.

Then there is this other thing.

Creation saw cause to implant a realm of consciousness that is real but imperceptible to the senses. Why? You tell me.

We choose to call this realm the unconscious. Why? Because we are informed that this realm exists when we are not awake! "One of the ways, of course, that we know of the existence of this vast but hidden realm of the mind...is through our dreams," wrote M. Scott Peck in The Road Less Traveled.

Peck elaborates by drawing a circle for a client and then placing a niche along the outer circumference, and then pointing to the small niche, saying, "That represents your conscious mind." He goes on to explain that all the remaining vastness of the circle represents the unconscious mind. That unconscious part of the mind we know nothing of; it is a part of us that we are entirely ignorant of. Yet if a person was to work hard and long enough to gain the knowledge contained in the unconscious mind, one would find "riches beyond imagination."

The awareness recovery journey is concerned primarily with the niche mentioned above. That niche - the conscious mind - is all you need to gain control of to stay sober. The irony, enigma, or paradox is that to know and control your conscious mind, you must become aware of and acknowledge that the unconscious exists, and realize it influences and informs your consciousness.

We can learn as much from the unconscious as from the senses of sight, touch, taste, smell, and sound if we seek it. When a person seriously takes this as a life purpose, they embark on the path to wisdom and enlightenment. This is certainly not meant for most of us to pursue in this lifetime. Who would make our French fries? But tapping into the knowledge that is unknown by the five conscious senses is done to gain the information stored there, and this the way to higher consciousness. Now, with that attainment, you can control your niche of the mind.

"Know thyself" are two words attributed to Socrates, an ancient philosopher of Greece. It does seem that knowing oneself is very important. What follows are suggestions for activities that will allow you to get acquainted with your body and mind and, consequently, your spiritual connection with the

Source/Universe - your own God consciousness.

YOGA

The benefit of Yoga is similar to meditation, but offers physical toning of the body and improves posture. You will quit slouching. Yoga reduces stress, increases energy, and elevates your mood. There are many types of Yoga. Do not concern yourself with one form being too strenuous. Find a Yoga that accommodates you. I found the following types of Yoga listed at one school: Hatha, Vinyasa, Kundalini, Sadhana, prenatal, postnatal, and restorative.

The following excerpt comes from the article "History of Yoga: A Complete Overview of the Yoga History," written by Shaynebance.

The saying, "What's in the past, should stay in the past," - doesn't work here.

We might already have an idea of what Yoga is, but to understand it better, we have to know what it has become as well as its roots and beginnings. A quick look at the history of Yoga will help us appreciate its rich tradition, and who knows, it might help us incorporate Yoga into our lives.

Although Yoga is said to be as old as civilization, there is no physical evidence to support this claim. Earliest archaeological evidence of Yoga's existence could be found in stone seals that depict figures of Yoga Poses. The stone seals place Yoga's existence around 3000 B.C.

Scholars, however, have a reason to believe that Yoga existed long before that and traced its beginnings in Stone Age Shamanism. Both Shamanism and Yoga have similar characteristics, particularly in their efforts to improve the human condition at that time. Also, they aim to heal community members, and the practitioners act as religious mediators. Though we know Yoga as focusing more on the self, it started out as community-ori-ented before it turned inward.

You may want to begin exercising, learning Tai Chi, or

practicing yoga after your morning meditation.

WALKING

Walking is a natural pace for humans. Running and even bicycling are normal, natural speeds. Once you begin moving over forty miles per hour, you are creating unnatural stress on your body and MSP. The thing that happens when you are walking is you have the luxury of pausing at will. When your curiosity is perked, you can stop and look at the details of the garden or listen to the dragonfly wings. Walking, even when you are in a hurry, gives you more control than driving. Stopping, slowing down, and speeding up are your decisions to make and not the force of the flow of the traffic.

When moving slower, you can turn around at will. You can take a small side street and discover a garden or, a park, or a bakery you never knew existed.

Walking is fun.

WRITING

Have you ever heard of a love letter? Do people write them anymore? We have become familiar with the phrase hate mail, but not love mail.

Writing is a way to express your feelings and get emotions out into the open. This is a cleansing and chakra-clearing activity. Therefore, journal writing is encouraged. A diary, a dream journal, or gratitude lists are ways to make writing a routine. If you are frustrated and angry about an issue, write about it. Put it down on paper and I promise you will be surprised how often your intuition bubbles a viable solution to you through the process. It is an activity that supports psychological and spiritual health.

Write a love letter.

DANCING

Dancing free is fun too. The great thing, someone pointed out to me, is that when you dance, you are not concerned about where you are going. Ballet, in contrast, does require precise knowledge of where the dancer will conclude a dance, but it's the much-heightened awareness required that is conscious-ness-raising and spiritually beneficial.

DRAWING/PAINTING/SCULPTING

Anyone can draw. Anyone can paint or even sculpt clay. Have you ever doodled while talking on the phone or while listening to a lecture? Doodling is drawing. The benefits of drawing include improving creativity, improving memory, and honing problem-solving. Drawing can be a great stress reducer, and it is also great at increasing awareness.

The drawing's details and specifics of the subject are closely examined and carefully and very consciously observed.

HOBBY

Knitting and sewing are serene pastimes. So are doing jigsaw puzzles, or building model cars, planes, or trains. These are hobbies that can have the same benefits as those mentioned above of drawing.

READING

Reading educates and opens the mind. It allows discovery and exploration. Through reading one can expand the possibilities of imagination. In all my research for this book and years of study in sub-jects from art to mythology, bathroom plumbing to zoology, it has never been suggested to increase my television viewing hours. TV programming is, after all, programming you.

MEDITATION

The human mind is capable of limitless expansion.

The mind-soul-psyche has infinite potential.

When the topic of meditation comes up, many people immediately revolt, "I cannot stop my mind from thinking!" Sure, you can. What you call thinking is not really thinking - it is worrying. Allowing random thoughts to roll, aimless and relentless, in your mind is not thinking. When you are not in control of your thoughts, you are hardly being thoughtful.

Meditation is easy. Think of it as a long bathroom break. Sit down, get comfortable, relax while your feet are flat on the floor, and focus your mind on something you will never see. The longer you are there, the more satisfying are the results.

Random thought will come and go white you attempt to meditate. That's okay. Return your focus to what you will never see.

People who claim they cannot control how they feel are also incapable of controlling what they think. Psychologist, physician, and philosopher William James said, "A great many people think they are thinking when they are merely rearranging their prejudices."

Think about that!

Phil Jackson, NBA champion head coach, described his meditation in an interview as surrendering the self to gravity.

Meditation will help you learn to think because you will learn mind control. It will help you be aware of your thoughts and control them.

Thinking is putting thoughts to reach a conclusion not known before. That is the only way to have an original thought. Most of the time, people are thinking similarly. That's why we exclaim, "Hey! I thought of that before!" Someone said something about something you had thought earlier and someone you don't know thought it before you did. Common thoughts are in the ether of the Universe.

We need quiet time to rest. Our brains, nerves, and every part of our bodies grow weary. Resting is different than sleeping. Sleep has its place for certain. But during the day, unless we are bedridden or in a drunken, drugged stupor, our bodies and brains need a break. This is how we eliminate stress.

Meditation makes you aware of you, Rebecca Rosen, psychic to the stars (celebrities) and author of Spirited, has these suggestions. She calls them "Easy-Peasy Meditations." If you have never learned to meditate, consider these activities.

While I do not agree these are meditation practices, I do agree they bring serenity to the soul and focus for the mind's attention. I have taken the liberty to rephrase Rosen's five "easy-peasy" meditations.

GO OUTSIDE AND BREATHE! Hold your head up and breathe the air deeply. This is great in cool weather. Turn your face to the sun when it is shining. Soak in that good and nutritious energy.

TAKE A SOAKING SCENTED BATH! Why not?

This is recommended by author and energy healer Deborah King. To be done frequently with sea salt and baking soda for clearing chakras.

USE YOUR KITCHEN! Make a fruit salad. Make a green salad. Learn to make bread and make a loaf; knead the dough with a complete focus on kneading.

LISTEN TO MUSIC THAT SOOTHES! Find a musical genre that is soothing to your soul.

Preferably without lyrics, as the words will distract you from yourself and shift attention and focus to another's past life experience. That is what lyrics to a song are: another soul's experience in life.

MOVE! Walk around the block to take a break instead of pacing to and from, directionless. Dance around the room without care of anything.

Easy-peasy meditations are great ways to relieve temporary stress from daily routines.

Try a ten-minute meditation in a more traditional manner. With eyes closed, seated in a comfortable position, and your focus on breathing and heartbeat. When really focusing on breathing or your heartbeat, it is easier to not think of other crap and still your mind.

The news to you may be to learn that meditation is necessarily to empty your mind. You are learning to control your mind. Keeping your body still is learning to control your body's actions.

The following statement is taken from how-to-meditate.org: "By training in meditation, we create an inner space and clarity that enables us to control our mind regardless of the external circumstances.

Gradually, we develop mental equilibrium, a balanced mind that is happy all the time, rather than an unbalanced mind that oscillates between the extremes of excitement and despondency."

As daily meditation becomes habit, what happens is that you increase your awareness and alertness throughout the day. You start to enjoy this heightened state of consciousness. You find it a superb replacement for mind-altered and addled oblivion.

Beginning quiet meditation requires silent stillness. The first thing for some of you to do that may be very difficult is turn off the phone.

Then turn off everything else!

Use an egg timer or a guided meditation that has ten, fifteen, or twenty minutes of music or spoken instruction. Mind Valley Academy usually has free downloads online.

Sit down and just listen to the silence or your choice of audio.

It may take weeks, even if you do this every day, but eventually, the chatter in your mind will slow balanced mind that is happy all the time, rather than an unbalanced mind that oscillates between the extremes of excitement and despondency."

As daily meditation becomes a habit, what happens is that you increase your awareness and alertness throughout the day. You start to enjoy this heightened state of consciousness. You find it a superb replacement for mind-altered and addled oblivion.

Beginning quiet meditation requires silent stillness. The first thing for some of you to do that may be very difficult is turn off the phone.

Then turn off everything else!

Use an egg timer or a guided meditation that has ten, fifteen, or twenty minutes of music or spoken instruction. Mind Valley Academy usually has free downloads online.

Sit down and just listen to the silence or your choice of audio.

It may take weeks, even if you do this every day, but eventually, the chatter in your mind will slow down. It will know from habit that you want it to get peaceful. So, don't worry. Progress will be made with habitual practice.

One thing that is always stressed in meditation is breathing. Breathe deeply through your nose and fill up and exhale through your mouth. And fill up your lungs so that your stomach, not your chest, expands.

Through meditation, intuitive insight will become dependable. You will come to dream reality. You will create your own reality, just as you did under the influence of mind-altering drugs; only this time, you will manifest healthy, sober dreams, objectives, and ultimate goals.

The Silva Life System has training in many aspects of meditation. The author and psychic mentioned earlier, Rebecca Rosen, does as well in Spirited: Connect to the Guides All Around You.

Anytime your mind is focused on one task, a form of meditation takes place. When thoughts are focused and we are finding pleasure and contentment, we are reducing stress. Here are a few other activities I consider meditative.

"Three Simple Ways Meditation Will Make You a Better Entrepreneur" is an article written by entrepreneur Russell Simmons and posted online in Entrepreneur magazine. Here are excerpts from that article.

"Meditation is going to make you happier and more connected to the world. That's what it's done for me, and that makes it the most beautiful gift that I could share with any of you."

"It's also the most effective tool to help you achieve your higher goals."

"When you sit quietly and let your mind settle, all the innovative, inventive, and inspired ideas that have been hiding out in the depths of your mind are going to begin to bubble to the surface."

"If, like most of us, you haven't been blessed with the same gift for connecting with that creativity, you can use meditation to get there. I promise that if you meditate twice a day for twenty minutes for just six weeks, you will see incredible returns on that investment!"

"No matter what you do, or no matter how busy you perceive yourself to be, carve out 40 minutes a day for meditation. I promise you it will not only make you a better entrepreneur, but a better and healthier person as well."

Use an alarm clock, an egg timer, or a CD with a guided meditation to keep time. Sit straight but comfortably. Focus your attention on breathing in through your nose. Fill up your belly, not your chest, and exhale through your mouth. Whew. Keep your focus on your breath. When your mind drifts to another subject, return your attention to your breathing.

Baby steps are how we learn to walk. Begin with the ten minutes in the morning and once again in the afternoon or evening. Then increase that ten minutes to twenty minutes, as Simmons recommends.

Think about how often you pace the floor wondering what to do, or mindlessly looking at websites or television programs. That time will be much more wisely used in meditation.

Morality and Ethics

*"The greatness of a man is not in how much wealth he acquires,
but in his integrity and his ability to affect those around him positively."*

BOB MARLEY, Singer and songwriter

ONE OF THE GREATEST BENEFITS of sober living
is that there is no longer doubt about what you are doing
presently or what you did the day before. There is considerably
more self-mind control and emotional stability. There is
confidence that the correct action is being or has been taken.
There is no questioning of thoughts. Intuition is increasingly
reliable. Your hunch was right (about whatever). There is
certainty now that the next action taken will be right: accurate,
and agreeable to others. No harm to others or self is being
done, and no fear of a future with damaging consequences
exists.

Sober living means truthful living and keeps the
conscience free and clear, and at peace.

Excellence of thought and excellence of character;
Aristotle philosophized that these are the two different kinds
of human excellence that exist. This excellence in quality of
character is acquired by applying one's self fully to their
attainment. Honest appraisal of one's own character is
challenging, but is an opportunity to clean house. Building
character that is desirable is done by discovering what is
lacking.

Do you practice sufficient self-control to be considered a
person of restraint? For most people, we can restrict our
appetite for only some, a small portion of life's pleasures. The
condition that is true for alcoholics and addicts is that excess
of anything and everything is most usually common. Substance
abusers are greedy by definition.

Greed is a character trait that most assuredly needs
deconstruction to make one's personality desirable. This can
be achieved by curtailing the desire to have everything and ask

149

for more. Becoming more self-aware of our thoughts, we can catch the greedy thought before we go into the action of self-gratification.

Awareness of our actions increases with sobriety. We have an excellent opportunity while in treatment to gain that sort of self-awareness. Monitor our urges to fulfill cravings. Avoid temptation by choosing not to put our self in scenarios that offer temptation. We know we are weak to temptation.

Do we extend ourselves to help others who are in need have a better day? Or are we selfish and miserly with our time and energy? Addicts are usually too concerned with own affairs to be charitable in any way, shape, or form. Our pride tells us that someone else will do the work for us. We rationalize this because we claim no one lifted us up, and then this other person can do the same and lift themselves up. We forget that no one put us down into the conditions that required we be lifted up. We think we are doing all right. Our standards have sunk to such lows that we say with pride, "I have never been to jail." How totally ignorant is that? We are not supposed to go to jail in the first place. Or other cases, certain individuals will boast of the time they did time in the "big house" and show off their ink.

Being too lazy to expend our own energy for the betterment of another human is more than likely the alcoholic and addict's response to charitable deeds. This character flaw will noticeably change as we gain sobriety because we will feel guilt of conscience. This is a feeling we do not find pleasing.

To make ourselves feel good, we find that giving is better than receiving for the first time ever.

As these personality flaws are found and potentially corrected by abstinence from alcohol and drugs, because clarity of mind increases us up, and then this other person can do the same and lift themselves up. We forget that no one put us down into the conditions that required we be lifted up. We think we are doing all right. Our standards have sunk to such lows that we say with pride, "I have never been to jail." How totally ignorant is that? We are not supposed to go to jail in the first place. Or other cases, certain individuals will boast of the time they did time in the "big house" and show off their ink.

Being too lazy to expend our own energy for the betterment of another human is more than likely the alcoholic and addict's response to charitable deeds. This character flaw will noticeably change as we gain sobriety because we will feel guilt of conscience. This is a feeling we do not find pleasing.

To make ourselves feel good, we find that giving is better than receiving for the first time ever.

As these personality flaws are found and potentially corrected by abstinence from alcohol and drugs, because clarity of mind increases awareness, we also find a slightly lifted spirit residing in our expression that is beneficial to self-esteem. We see that our actions of love for others and respect for our own lives through temperance and moderation satisfies our souls. We begin to feel good about our self and enjoy the growing respectability we are achieving amongst society.

Our demeanor is changing. We can look straight ahead on the street and at others directly in the eyes. Our confidence is strengthening. Our self-esteem continues to rise. We feel good, and we like it. We can see loving ourselves, instead of feeling shameful about our actions; we now sense real pride instead of false arrogance, conceit, and egotism.

We begin to seek where we can be helpful more and more to others. Morality, we are coming to understand, is on display in how we conduct ourselves.

Some things are easy to repair. Improving morality is not, but we accept the challenge, as we saw an opportunity to improve the quality of our own life. Our motivation was selfish, but it was in the pursuit of positive energy being sent and received.

Whatever it is you don't like about yourself will haunt you if not corrected. Many things we make harder to correct than is necessary. Because we have courageously begun this new path in life, change has come to us. Change in principles, values, and behavior is finding us reborn.

We are learning about our good self. We see now that an unfavorable outer condition, like a job or a marriage, that makes us unhappy can be corrected, improved, or dismissed by our own authority. We no longer procrastinate but instead tackle problems directly.

Allowing undesirable conditions to persist really does ferment and spoil and rot our soul. And this we find no longer an acceptable life experience.

We have found that by addressing the problem, we are crafting a positive outlook and taking a healthy stance.

Matters of conscience prevail and triumph when honesty and truthfulness overcomes, and overrides deceit and lies.

Universally, philosophies have defined high moral standards. The ethical virtues found preferable are many but vary very little, considering the diversity of human societies from Aruba to Zimbabwe, Arizona to Sweden. Love and kindness are a constant.

Galatians 5:22-23 from the New International

Version Bible reads, "But the fruit of the Spirit is love, joy, peace, forbearance (leniency/mercy), kindness, goodness, faithfulness, gentleness and self-control. Against such things, there is no law."

The principles that guide the Twelve Steps of AA are honesty, hope, faith, courage, integrity, willingness, humility, reflection, forgiveness, acceptance, spirituality, and service.

A person with self-control, discipline, is universally admired. Self-discipline is extremely important for substance abusers to acquire.

Awareness recovery aims to elevate one's consciousness to the extent that over-indulgence becomes appalling. Acting without restraint from pursuing passionately the thoughtless, careless whims of years past appears deliberately frivolous.

This higher quality of character is what we need to say, "No, I don't want a drink. I have had enough. Thanks." And right there, in that statement, honesty and courage are demonstrated.

Place discipline, honesty, and courage on your list of ethical qualities you wish to attain through daily practice. Write these three attributes in your journal. Writing reinforces objectives in our consciousness.

Consider the principles that you admire and would like to model. When people think of you, what words do they use? Ask someone, "How would you describe me?" You may be surprised by what three different people will tell you. Ask, "What is the first word that comes to mind when you think of me?"

If pimp, slutty, mean, grumpy, devilish, angry, jealous, scary, stupid-in-a-good-way, or asshole is used, then add these to your list of personality flaws. Then consider how to correct specifically the outward image people see. Certainly, we do not want to continue life known as that "scary bitch" or "stingy old bastard."

Write in your journal thoughts about what you see in yourself. Don't be afraid to ask a counselor, "What is your impression of me?"

A counselor may well see through the character that we portray to the public because they have spoken in private and confidential circumstances with us. The counselor may, in fact, reward us with encouragement by offering up the potential strengths of character they have perceived underneath the armor and shield we carry to battle in defense of our frail ego.

"You really are an intelligent person; have you considered returning to school to get a degree or professional certification in the future?" That is the question the counselor posed when you are expected to hear, "You seem bright. What else do you want?" But with consideration of the future as an intelligent and sober person, you are asked to dig deeper inside for a response. That is good. It means you have a good addictions counselor.

Appearance does make a difference in the way other people respond to you. The same way you are making changes to your moral character, you want to consider making changes to wardrobe, hairstyle, and hygiene. "Image is everything" was a slogan popularized by eight-time Grand Slam champion Andre Agassi.

The goal is to become attractive inside and out.

To be a person to whom people are attracted instead of repelled by.

We do not, by any means, want to dress the part of a gentleman or lady and remain a wolf inside.

Not by any means are we going to retain that boastful, load-mouthed persona that once cloaked our frightened, insecure alcoholic/addict self. What is the opposite of the stuck-up, phony, and arrogant person we are leaving behind? A person willing to learn generosity, humility, and kindness is our conclusion.

Write generosity, humility, and kindness in your journal. Consider ways to incorporate these admirable ethical and moral characteristics into your life. Using the courage that you have already determined worthy to cultivate, consider doing something you have never done. Volunteer at a hospital, school, housing shelter, food pantry, or church, or offer housekeeping or transportation to the physically disadvantaged or mentally challenged. Any of these activities would certainly address becoming humble, kind, and generous simultaneously. And you are being of service to the community and society at large as opposed to being an ever-threatening menace.

Shifting lust for fulfilling our vain pleasures to lust for sharing love, joy, and peace to others has been and is now and will continue, daily, to be our focus. This is where our attention has been turned, and our intention pointed. Gentleness and goodness could not help but follow us on our path to integrity.

Being at peace within ourselves makes working with others, whether paid or voluntary, easy. It is no longer a burden to be reliable.

Acceptance, patience, and tolerance are three moral virtues if we learn to exercise patience. Patience is a very difficult virtue for addictive personalities. The overwhelming urge for instant gratification has been cemented firmly in many of us. Patience takes time to learn. The benefit of being a patient person is that frustration over simple everyday occurrences will not throw us into a boiling rage of horrendous verbal abuse or demented demonstrations of violence. Patience circumvents anger and fury. Practiced daily, perhaps by simply taking time to pause before speaking, breathe before acting, patience inevitably results in our gaining tolerance for others and acceptance of circumstances.

Forgiveness and faithfulness are possibly the two characteristics of ethical, moral fiber that a substance abuser is completely unfamiliar with in actions and attitude. Be sure to write these virtues in your exit strategy journal.

Faithfulness: a promise of fidelity. The word "faithful" has many synonyms, each of which stirs a variety of subtle nuances in every individual's response. Some cringe at and some wistfully long for the experience of faithfulness. Being faithful is most often linked in our culture to the intimate partnership of romance and fiscal moderation.

Loyalty comes to mind immediately, doesn't it? Okay. What next? Commitment! Yes, to be faithful requires commitment, and what else? How about trustworthiness? Trust is very important. That is the foundation of being faithful. That's good. Reliability and dependability are also expected in a contract of faithfulness. This next word is probably expected least, and that is why it is mentioned last. The word is devotion. Who even uses that word anymore? What is it? Many will ask this, bewildered, and are thrown into an intellectually incomprehensible roadblock, mental jam, and utter cerebral quandary over the simple word "devotion."

155

Devotion to anyone or any institution means to express affection, willingness to care, dedication to the mission, and fondness for forever. This is ultimately all faithfulness. Handle it. Or better yet, accept it.

Families shatter like glass on stone, break up like porcelain thrown upon marble, and burn like paper in an inferno in the face of unfaithfulness. Some of us already know this, but a reminder never does any harm.

Forgiveness is an act of love. It is the act of forgiving. When we forgive, we give up resentment of something said or done that was offensive.

Whether the offense was intentional or incidental, even malicious or only accidental, the person perpetuating the insult is freed from penalty or retribution.

We will want to forgive ourselves and will want to ask forgiveness from others when we are ready.

"I forgive you; I won't hate you always. You are forgiven," is often said to rectify infidelity. Apologies gush like a geyser to repair a betrayal, like when sexual relations happen outside of a marriage without the partner's consent: meaning a cheating, deceitful extra-marital affair has come to light. Houses have been burnt to the ground due to this treacherous liaison.

To really get into the complexity of forgiveness, there is one book strongly recommended. Reverend Tutu has forgiven entire nations and races of people for injustices. He knows a lot about the subject.

Archbishop Emeritus of Cape Town, the Most Reverend Desmond Tutu, co-authored with his daughter, Reverend Mpho Tutu, The Book of Forgiving. If you want to study exercises in forgiving, how to forgive and how to accept forgiveness, this is a workbook for practicing and learning this moral virtue.

The full title of this man is given here to honor the tremendous service Reverend Tutu has given to the entire world as a diplomat and social activist in bringing peace and understanding to peoples in conflict over issues of apartheid, terrorism, and equal rights for all peoples, regardless of race, sexuality, or gender. Tutu is deemed and revered as "South Africa's moral conscience."

Do you seek to live honestly? Are you ready to live legally in society? Can you be worthy of trust? Do you consistently fulfill obligations? Can you be competent and industrious? Can you be fair and generous in your interactions with others? Do you want to live life with self-control, kindness, and tolerance?

Saying yes, to any of the above, is the correct answer.

Drug-free living brings clarity of mind and a clear conscience. Living in such a manner can only bring a productive and trouble-free life. Of course, there will be challenges and difficulties, but sober, we can address the problem instead of drinking and sinking, doping, and hoping life goes away.

For being competent and industrious in life, happiness and prosperity will be your reward. Remember to do no harm to self or others, and do not do to another person or any animal anything that...well, we know the Golden Rule saying is to do to others as you would have them do to you - something like that, but presented here with a positive spin.

No matter how self-involved and narcissistic we have been, now we see, with open hearts and open minds, that there are better ways to behave and live human.

Live and Learn

"Food for the body is not enough. There must be food for the soul."

- **DOROTHY DAY**, American journalist, social activist

LEARNING TO MAKE WISE DECISIONS and follow through with correct actions is important. This is because bad decisions, 99.9% of the time, cost more grief, money, and/or time than the issue of the situation was worth. We are responsible for our experience in life. For instance, a policeman pulls you over in your car or while walking. You can be amicable, courteous, and compliant and drive or walk away free (or possibly with a warning from the lawman).

You can also be angry, unruly, and argumentative and be thrown to the ground, handcuffed, and taken to jail.

Is being belligerent worth the ruination of your plans for the day?

Your intuition should instantly say no. Don't react foolishly. That is precisely what the lawman wants. Never let pride override good sense. Your mission is too valuable to be interrupted and sidetracked by the powers that be.

Stand up for your rights only when provoked.

Always remain calm. De-escalate the confrontation with reasonableness. Do not play into the hand of law enforcement. Many officers are hopped up and easily excitable. There are many possible reasons, like steroid use, social prejudices, poor attitude, general anger, not meditating in the morning.

What follows are true stories of bad decisions.

JAYWALKING

A woman was jogging with her earplugs in her ears, listening to something she enjoyed. This was where her focus was. She jaywalked, jogging across a street. A policeman shouted, "Hey! Stop!" trying to get the jogger to stop to ticket her. The jogger remained oblivious. She did not hear the officer and continued to jog along the sidewalk. The policeman was infuriated! He chased her down, dropped her to the ground, and handcuffed the bewildered jogger, and the young lady was taken to jail. It's on video!

How many bad decisions were made in this scenario?

RESISTING ARREST

This story has so many bad decisions, you pick one. A middle-aged woman, drunk on beers, kicked the policeman attempting to arrest her for public intoxication and destruction of private property. She was trying to break into her estranged husband's home to see her daughter.

The officer completed the arrest. The charge of public intoxication did not get her three years in prison. Kicking the cop did. Public intoxication, resisting arrest, and assaulting an officer was the case before the judge. The judge looked at her record. This was not the first time this woman had assaulted an officer. The judge looked at the middle-aged, 5'2", maybe 120-pound woman and decided she was a danger to society and sentenced her to three years in state prison (no time off for good behavior).

TAKING SHORTCUTS

The biggest blunder I ever heard was a man that thought he could use a Kirtland Air Force base as a shortcut to drive to the other side of town to get donuts for his wife. Military police pulled him over after he passed by the guard gate and arrested him.

They had him handcuffed in their jeep while they were searching his vehicle. The donut man escaped the handcuffs, started the police jeep, and took off in it.

Nine years was the sentence he was handed.

When asked what he was doing time for, he always answered, "Donuts."

DISOBEYING LAW ENFORCEMENT

Brian Encinia, a Texas state trooper, pulled behind Sandra Bland while she was driving in the left-hand lane. A state trooper behind me always makes me nervous, so I assume Sandra was too when she saw the vehicle behind her was a state trooper. She directed her vehicle into the right-hand lane, I can only guess to let the law enforcement officer pass.

The report from Officer Brian Encinia is that she failed to signal a lane change with her blinker and, so he was justified in pulling her over.

Officer Encinia approached the driver-side window and asked her to roll the window down.

Rumor is that Sandra had smoked marijuana in her car very recently, and that is why Sandra refused to roll the window down. She wanted to know, speaking through the rolled-up window, why she had been stopped. This went on for a few minutes, exasperating any patience the officer had, and he began demanding she step out of the car. Allegedly, a scuffle ensued that was initiated by Sandra's unwillingness to comply once she was out of the vehicle.

The excerpt below was taken from an article in the Huffington Post. The end results of the Sandra

Brown arrest were:

WALLER COUNTY, TEXAS - On July 13, (2015)

Sandra Bland, a 28-year-old black woman, was found dead in her jail cell in Waller County, Texas, three days after being arrested over a traffic stop gone wrong. Sheriff Glenn Smith, who oversees the county jail and had been fired from a previous job after allegations of racism and police brutality, promised an all access, top-to-bottom investigation to uncover what happened to Bland. He set up an "independent" commission to review the sheriff's department. Smith tapped Paul Looney, a local criminal defense lawyer, to lead the probe and to pick the commission's other members.

The "story" is that after three days in the county jail,

Sandra Bland was able to hang herself with a trash bag in a suicide.

Sheriff Smith, a suspected racist (see allegations in the above excerpt), and a defense lawyer named Looney began a probe into this "suicide" of an incarcerated inmate.

They must use Hefty trash bags in Waller County's jail to carry all the manure in that place.

OPEN CONTAINER

A driver made an illegal left turn on Sunset Boulevard in Hollywood, California, on a dark winter's evening, and a police officer pulled him over. He complied courteously with the officer and explained he was lost. The policeman gave him directions but not a ticket, and before the officer walked back to his patrol car, he said, "Don't spill your beer on the floor behind you."

Certainly, if this driver had been belligerent with the officer on Sunset Boulevard, he would have been taken in for the open bottle of beer in his vehicle. Luckily for the driver, it was Hollywood, and the police have much more to do than deal with open beer bottles. Still, it was a bad decision to open the forty-ounce bottle in the car.

DRINKING AND DRIVING

The judge's sentence was six months' probation for Dave's first DUI (Driving Under the Influence). His last words to Dave and his attorney were, "If you are ever in a Maryland court again, you'll do three months' minimum jail time."

Dave never forgot that.

The events leading up to the DUI mentioned involved a company Christmas party with an open bar. The celebration took place in a large hotel ballroom with more than a hundred employees and perhaps as many clients. The round tables were elegantly dressed in white tablecloths and napkins and complete formal settings of silverware. Each table was set for twelve. Dave and his best co-worker friend, Pete, took seats together. Their conversation turned to popular music. They knew no one else at the table, but when they agreed that the music of Barry Manilow was terrible, a large, red-faced, heavy-set man with gray hair spoke up.

"My son is Manilow's music director."

Oops! Pete and Dave changed the topic of their conversation.

The party ended, and Dave headed home. It was not yet midnight when, turning the corner about a mile from home, Dave fell asleep at the wheel. When he woke up, he was sitting on the ceiling of the car. The radio was playing loudly. He turned the volume knob in one direction, and the music got loud. Because he was upside down, turning the knob left or right had the opposite response.

The results were that the vehicle was totaled.

The ambulance and the police arrived. When asked if he needed medical attention, Dave declined, and the police took him into custody.

The six months' probation required that Dave report every Tuesday to an office, fill out a form, and wait until the probation officer said he could leave. Being that alcohol was Dave's only vice and probation visits were on Tuesdays, he drank Thursday, Friday, Saturday, and Sunday. He abstained Monday, Tuesday, and sometimes Wednesday. The six months passed painlessly and unthreateningly.

Time went by and a year passed without a driving or drinking incident.

Monday-night football was popular at the time, and Dave went to a friend's house with a pint of Scotch.

As he returned home on the highway, flashing lights came on behind him. He was in Maryland. The judge had said he'd do jail time if ever brought into court again for drinking and driving. He was about ten miles from the state line. If he could get into Virginia before being pulled over, then he would not be in Maryland.

Dave stepped on the gas. When he got to the last exit and entrance ramp in Maryland there were five state troopers waiting. Dave sped through them. They fell in behind him. At ninety miles an hour, Dave led the state troopers on what is called a rolling roadblock. Desperately, they tried to stop Dave before he got to Virginia. Just as he crossed into Virginia, a Maryland state trooper pulled in front of Dave and stopped. Dave stomped on his brakes.

Virginia state troopers had heard of the pursuit. They were waiting. While Dave was lying face down on the highway, the state troopers from Maryland and Virginia argued over custody. The Maryland officers lost. Dave won.

He went to a Virginia jail for the night.

ADDICT WITH ACCESS

Tribune-Review/Pittsburgh Tribune-Review

DOCTOR ADDICTED TO VICODIN, FEDS SAY By Bowling, Brian

A prominent doctor facing 185 federal charges that include drug trafficking is addicted to the narcotic painkiller Vicodin, a federal prosecutor said Monday.

To feed his habit, Dr. Richard A. Rydze, 62, of the Strip District forged prescriptions in another doctor's name and issued them to Rydze's deceased father, said Special Assistant U.S. Attorney Carol Skutnik.

U.S. Magistrate Judge Robert Mitchell released Rydze -- a former doctor for the Pittsburgh Steelers and the FBI's field office on home confinement with a $100,000 unsecured bond and ordered Rydze to surrender his prescription pads.

"He's not going to work," the judge said. "He's going to stay home."

Skutnik urged Mitchell to keep Rydze in jail while he awaits trial because he continued to traffic in human growth hormones, anabolic steroids, and painkillers after agents twice raided his medical office and the Drug Enforcement

Administration suspended his ability to prescribe drugs.

Before the second raid, he gathered patient records and began altering them to hide what he was doing, she said.

"He has thumbed his nose at this investigation," Skutnik said.

Assistant Federal Public Defender Marketa Sims argued that Rydze has ties to the community and showed no intent to flee even though he knew investigators were watching him since 2007. She did not address whether he's an addict.

"Everything he cares about is here -- his wife, his kids, his practice," Sims said.

We create our reality. We are responsible for every step we take and, every word we say, how we walk, and how we talk. Bad decisions never bring good outcomes.

We have choices about what we experience. We have choices about the knowledge we wish to attain and retain. Therefore, when we love ourselves, we make wiser decisions for our safety and experience more positive results, and one happy day after another becomes, at best, routinely normal.

Sacred Cow

Meditation is probably the single best thing you can do for your physical, mental, and spiritual health. It stills the mind, relaxes the body, and cleans your chakras. The benefits of meditation have recently been proven by science, but have been known to humans for centuries. Nearly every culture throughout human history has used some form of med-itation to achieve a variety of enhancements such as: stress-reduction; increases in focus and memory; decreases in muscle tension, cholesterol, and heart rate; enhanced immune system function, athletic performance, and weight loss; better sleep and the need for less of it, and so many more. Meditation has even been shown to be more effective than prescrip-tion drugs in lowering anxiety and depression.

Now, you will receive some of these benefits doing any type of meditation, but if you learn meditation correctly from an experienced instructor or spiritual teacher, the benefits multiply to include higher levels of conscious-ness, better connection to Source, and a boost to your spiritual journey.

Belief that your body is a sacred temple will go a long way in raising your consciousness, dignity and self-awareness.

An acquaintance from Nepal reminded me that the cow is sacred in Hindu and not to be eaten.

They eat goats and sheep. He told me that in Hindu communities of Nepal, anyone killing a cow faces twenty years' imprisonment. The sanctity of a cow is difficult to understand in a country that markets cow meat with the slogan "Where's the beef?"

Religionfacts.com offers this clarification to the question "Why is the cow important to Hindus?"

In Hinduism, the cow is revered as the source of food (milk) and symbol of life and may never be killed. However,

165

many non-Hindus interpret these beliefs to mean that Hindus worship cows. This is not true. It is more accurate to say the cow is taboo in the Hindu religion, rather than sacred. This is just one example of the misunderstand-ings people have about the Hindu faith.

The cow remains a protected animal in Hinduism today and Hindus do not eat beef. Most rural In-dian families have at least one dairy cow, a gentle spirit who is often treated as a member of the family.

Don't you think the price of beef is expensive in the United States? Maybe cows ought to be taboo here too.

Seek the sacred and more is revealed. We see that life is a cycle and the cycle of life is blessed.

Everyone has something that they feel reverence toward. That something may gain their respect, it may be worthy of worship, or it may simply be highly admired. Is it sacred? Seeking the sacred usually finds us in agreement that life is sacred. Then we see the sacred that is in life. Everything that gives us life can be viewed sacred. Air, water, earth, and fire, which provides heat and the ability to cook foods that require cooking to purge it of things that will make us sick.

I believe nature is largely sacred. That might be what was meant when a band named itself Earth, Wind & Fire. There are also things in nature that are dangerous to life, which is why I can't perceive pests as sacred. Roaches, fleas, mosquitoes, and ticks cannot be revered in my worldview.

There are man-made sacred ceremonies, too. We consider marriage to be a sacred relationship. Baptism is a sacred ceremony. There are various sacred ceremonies throughout the myriad of world cultures. Some see certain stones as sacred. Though stone has no life as we know life to be, it exists. We may marvel at some aspect of it, its color or shape, as it captures our mind's attention.

In the sacred we may find God and Source.

I believe that what is sacred is something you can bring to mind for the purpose of aligning your inner-self and consciousness with positive energy when in prayer or meditation. Think of something you truly treasure.

This is positive thinking. This will help allay the fears or resentments you have regarding some matter over which you have no control and which is frustrating you to no end.

You want to get your mind correct and at peace before praying, meditating, or walking the dog. This is because if you continue to dwell in negativity, you will only receive negativity and step in your dog's poop.

Bob Marley sings in Positive Vibration, "If you get up and quarrel every day, you're saying prayers to the devil, I say."

Pause. Breathe. You don't have to be in AA to remember to HALT, which is an acronym to remind a person to never get too Hungry, Angry, Lonely, or Tired. Any of these conditions can ruin good vibes. And they can all be prevented, too.

Find a way to experience nature. If you live in a city, find a park and make it a ritual to routinely go there. Commune, communicate with nature. This activity assists us in being grounded, down to Earth. Being witness to the splendor of nature makes us pause to hold in reverence the miracle that surrounds us and is within us. We are humbled by the majesty that is creation. Walk in the park in awe and wonder at the grandeur of it all and the splendor of the smallest flower. Find a place to sit on the grass and lean your back against a tree. Look up and watch the leaves of the trees tremble in the slightest breeze, or the branches sway in a steady wind. Look down and watch the grass grow. Have no doubt each blade is growing. Close your eyes, breathe deeply through your nostrils, and exhale slowly through your lips, listening for the sound of "whew" as the air leaves your body, transformed from oxygen inhaled to carbon dioxide, which the trees and the grass will breathe before they exhale oxygen to sustain your living experience. Plants pull carbon dioxide from the air and convert it to oxygen, releasing the oxygen into the atmosphere (the ether). This is the cycle we share with the life of plants. The carbon dioxide produced within our human body in burning food for fuel energy escapes in exhalation into the ether with our breath.

Consider this cycle and the subtle silent sacredness that surrounds you, and embrace the stillness with all your senses. Some say the Judaic printed letters for God, YHWH, is the sound "whew" when we exhale a breath of air through our lips.

If you can go to a lake, a river, a seashore or ocean beach occasionally, do it, go there. Marvel at the ripples in a pond, the flow of a creek as water streams to a future unknown. Listen to the sound. Delight in the sight of waves coming to the shoreline of the coast in tides responding to the cycle of the moon. Listen to the sound of the waves crashing as they cause the sand to shift, sometimes slowly and sometimes suddenly. All in this environment is ever changing; know now that this is the same energy that causes change in you constantly. Go with the flow.

Bring a plant home and care for it. Some houseplants produce more oxygen than others. Ferns are good. The royal Japanese fern releases oxygen into the air and absorbs formaldehyde. The Boston fern adds oxygen and humidity to the air inside your office or home. Philodendrons and spider plants also produce great quantities of oxygen and are easy to care for while enhancing the symbiotic relationship that exists between animals and plants: two different kinds of living things living in the same space while depending on each other. If this is not unconditional love, then what is?

Adopt a pet and love it. Watch whichever you choose, be it plant or pet, as he or she grows in response to your careful attention. Witness and appreciate the response you have prompted by caring and observe your own soul's gratitude for the unconditional love that is shared between plant or pet and you.

Acknowledge that you prefer life this way. Consider the opposite. If you expressed no kindness and no generosity to the plant or pet, then you would certainly have a dying plant and a pet with an angry attitude.

If you are snowed in, build a fire for comfort or watch the snowfall from out the window for a while. Relax your mind. You are in control. Do not allow your mind to fret and worry or stew in useless aggravation. Quiet the noise. Let it rain, let it blossom, let it grow, and let it go.

"All things must pass." - **George Harrison.**

This is the same with our relationships and communication with people, places, and everything there is. "All our human relationships are secondary because they are bound by time and must pass away," writes Dr. David Frawley in Ayurveda and the Mind: The Healing of Consciousness. Frawley also states, "Our real relationship, which is eternal, is with the Divine."

Learn to practice patience and unconditional love.

Circumstances and conditions change constantly. Count your blessings, as they say. Be grateful—accept flow and flux as a gift. We should be happy that "shit" happens and that opportunities to challenge our mind, body, and spirit occur. The energy originates from the Source. We control our destiny.

This is a blessing, and your life is special and sacred.

And your earthly experience will end only to continue in the eternal ether as one energy with the Universe. There may not be an end for our energy spirit but only a transition to another realm of consciousness. And what if there never was a beginning? What if the Universe and you as energy has always and forever existed and only transforms and morphs according to cosmic law?

An indefinable mystery, a nebulous enigma, best describes God: The Source. In my imaginative hours of speculations on the mysteries of the universes, I came up with the following theosophy. Theosophy is any philosophy based on intuitive insight into the true nature of God. This is mine.

THE THEOSOPHY OF SOURCE THAT HAS NO SOURCE

All begins with Source. All and everything begins with the Source. In this theosophy Source exists without a Source. There is a Source without source.

Source is. Source is All Eternal Essence of Everlasting Spirit. Source emanates the energy and elements to the infinite ether of endless Heavens.

Vibrations create sound, and higher frequencies of sound tones manifest as Light.

Energy and Elements together form Force.

Force gives Form to Spheres, and Spheres created Cycles. Force becomes Frequency, and so Vibration becomes Sound.

And so, it is. An atom and its protons and neutrons are eternal. If split, they cause destruction to creation, and when brought together, they form reality as we see it. When all essence is eternal, such as all the atoms ever made are, would not this ultimately explain our ecstatic belief in and enthusiasm for eternal life?

This theosophy is best described in metaphor.

Human existence created by Source is subject to the cycles seen in the Spheres and heard in the Sound. And so, the Spirituality of humankind is like that of water.

The metaphor I make is that of a lake. A reservoir of humankind likened to the water of a lake. And there are a finite number of lakes, just as there are finite ethnicities and tribes. But when returned to the ether as water evaporated, all are one again.

Each human is but a droplet of the water in the lake. The water in the lake comes from the Source, which springs forth from groundwater below. Source is without Source because it recycles. Water from the ground goes up to the sky. And rain brings it back down to the ground.

No droplet is distinguishable or distinct from another until the journey begins. The journey begins with the formation of rivers and streams, brooks, and creeks flowing toward the ocean and sea. Water, once divided on the journey through rivers and streams, brooks and creeks, is reunited in the oceans and seas. The water is transformed over time, from the Energy of the Sun, to vapor.

Evaporation disperses the molecules of what will become clusters of vaporous clouds. The clouds then produce droplets of water as rain. Humankind is like the rain.

A raindrop falling is like the lifespan of a human in the eons of time beyond time. A human lifespan is smaller than a grain of sand. The time it takes for a raindrop to fall from the sky to the ground is all the time we will know ourselves as separate from the other: individuals.

The ground absorbs the water. And while some will return to the groundwater to go through the long cyclical journey to the spring to the lake to the rivers and streams, brooks and creeks, to the ocean and sea to the sky, some water will feed the green trees and other things that grow in color.

Imagine this analogy of humankind as water in the theosophy of Source without Source. This is a theosophy I originated to entertain and spark your imagination. We can believe anything. Humankind as water in relation to the unexplainable Source: God allows an imaginative glimpse into the duality in the oneness we perceive. We are immortal souls, one with God: The Source.

All is one.

From Dr. David Frawley: "The mind is a creation primarily of the ether element of Nature. In substance, the mind is like space - expansive, open, and all-pervading.... Ether exists in the mind as its underlying mind-space, the background capacity for all mental functions, vibrations, and impressions."

HONESTY

Would you say that learning to walk after age ten or eleven, given that there are no physical limitations, would be preposterous? Then maybe you would agree that learning ethical behavior, good moral character, and how to practice virtuous values after age seventeen is a damn shame.

Yet it happens. It happened to me. Once, in treatment, being asked to prioritize my values, I faltered by asking, "What kind of values?" It would have been kind if the counselor had given us a ten-minute presentation about what values were, so we (or at least I) could select three or four first to prioritize.

After that group session, a young man I'd made a friendly acquaintance came over to me, shaking his head, and said, "Man! She blew me away!"

"Yeah, man. I didn't know anything about any values. My values are like, one-hundred-dollar bill is first, then a fifty-dollar bill and on down the denominations...you know what I mean?"

"I am no better, bro, because I was thinking of color values! Like in color charts, hues, shades, and values!"

"What did you write down?"

"I wrote God is priority value number one."

He said, "Me too." And we gave each other a low-five.

"What do they mean when they ask, what color do you feel today?"

"No damn idea," my session friend replied.

How sad is that? Two adults, college-educated men, did not know what "values" meant in the world of behavioral psychology.

Now, we all know what values are. If you missed it in a previous chapter, more than twenty values of ethical and moral virtue are listed below again. Work with the values that you think need to be improved in your life.

These are love, joy, peace, forbearance (leniency/mercy), kindness, goodness, faithfulness, gentleness and self-control, honesty, hope, courage, integrity, willingness, humility, reflection, forgiveness, acceptance, spirituality, and service. Let's add gratitude, self-respect, and generosity.

Select the virtues that you believe will help you become a person of higher ethical character in the future. The more, the better, but certainly, there are some that you already possess.

Maybe even consider looking at the antonyms of the virtues that you select. The opposite of humility is arrogance. "Am I arrogant?" would be the question to ask. Or acceptance versus rejection, willingness versus reluctance, integrity versus dishonesty, and so forth. Courage against cowardice. Some of these are going to be hard to face with honesty regarding ourselves.

Some of us have lied, but will tell no one. No one is asking you to tell anyone but you. This is your exit strategy. What you write is personal and only serves to benefit you. Examine your past way of life. Examine the values that you can see now with a clear mind in which there once was flawed thinking.

Using your new attitude toward life, consider the higher standards you have set for yourself to write worthwhile and attainable goals. What have you decided to change about you? Think of characteristics and mannerisms. How have your thoughts been modified over the past weeks?

Has anything changed for you, or are you simply coasting, playing the "game" as you have in the past, and only anticipating your first drink or blunt upon release? In that case, write integrity and honesty in your journal as virtues that you sorely lack. Are you so vain that you will not help you get right on track? Then, write that you need to increase your humility. While you are at it, include courage, because if you are afraid to face you in the mirror, then cowardice is something you have in too great abundance.

Acknowledge your strengths and choose to develop them further. Admit your weaknesses and determine to strengthen them.

For example, one of your strengths might be that you are friendly and people like you. Maybe a sales career is more suitable because you'd be working with the public. A weakness you acknowledge is that you frequently exaggerate the truth. You are a liar. Being honest with your spouse or employer is a commitment you will make.

Thinking of three areas in which you can improve is not easy.

Use silence. One or two traits might easily come to mind, but how to develop these or correct them may take some time to contemplate. You have learned now that in silence, your intuition becomes more available. The best answer will come.

This personal improvement cannot be done with distractions. Turn off the phone and TV and let anyone (a roommate at the treatment center, children at home, a nosy spouse) know you need thirty minutes of quiet time alone.

A new life awaits you. Anything in your life that makes you unhappy can be eliminated. Relationships, housing, community, employment, career, and even health and appearance can be changed. Much like a hairstyle that doesn't work for you anymore, it can be changed. Growing new hair takes longer than cutting it off, but it could be worth the wait.

Be patient and thorough and on course.

DREAM CONSCIOUSNESS

Some believe that our soul consciousness leaves our bodies when we dream in our sleep. I find that hard to believe, if at all. What do you think? Does our subconscious really go to the places of other dimensions? Is that why what we experience stirs emotions and our thoughts? Is that why we can wake up in fear or horny?

Dreams are certainly mysterious. Make no mistake. Dreams are real.

Staying the course is something that Daniel of the Bible's Old Testament did to the highest degree. Daniel and his three companions kept their bodies clean and clear, and this, in turn, raised the level of their consciousness, as is exhibited in Daniel's ability to read another man's dream.

Daniel's ability to know and interpret dreams delighted King Nebuchadnezzar, who rewarded him handsomely. Daniel dreams, and sees the king's dream. This coincides with the theories presented in the next chapter that we share consciousnesses in the ether.

Daniel 2:27-28: "Daniel replied, 'No wise man,

enchanter, magician, or diviner can explain to the king the mystery he has asked about, but there is a God in heaven who reveals mysteries." This is all about dream consciousness. It goes on: "Your dream and the visions that passed through your mind as you lay on your bed are these: As you were lying there, O king, your mind turned to things to come and the revealing of mysteries..."

Dreams play a significant role for many key figures in the Bible. What follows next is a discussion of the consciousness that gives access to dreams and intuition.

Intuition From the Ether

"We are all sending out vibrations through our consciousness. We cannot see the waves of energy we are sending out into the Universe; what we do see are the results of what we are projecting."

THE RELATIONSHIP CODE, MARGARET MCCRAW

GOD OR NO GOD, REINCARNATION or karma, is destiny fated or chosen by free will? As in politics and religion, to each their own. Since that is the case, here I toss my speculative theory into the ring of fiery discourse.

The discussion that follows dabbles with the metaphysical: relating to the transcendent or to a reality beyond what is perceptible to the senses; relating to things that are thought to exist but that cannot be seen.

Instinct, hunches, and intuition cannot be seen any more than air, but they are often correct. Intuition can be developed. Then honesty will become a way of life, too. Living lies only leads to more lies and, clouds our perception, and creates drama. Drama can lead to relapse.

Live with daily optimism. This leads to an open mind. Live in the moment of now. Your awareness of the present is important. Also, be attentive to your dreams. Practicing this way of being you, along with meditation, affirmations, and/or daily affirmations, will bring strength to intuitive skills. This will lead to the right decisions and a lot less stress and worry.

You will instinctively know when someone tells you something, if it is truth. As it is written in Luke 17:21: "They can't say, 'Here it is!' or 'There it is!' You see, the Kingdom of God is within you."

Can it be said any plainer? The journey to knowledge is a journey within you. What does this mean? It means to follow the example that has been practiced throughout the world for many millennia. Apply meditation and prayer to your life.

We know it is true that the Kingdom of God is within us. Seeking outside of ourselves for communication with the Source is folly. It is an inside job. That is why we become silent in prayer. This is why we grow silent when we meditate. Silence is required for communication with the deep consciousness inside each of us. Silence is golden.

There exists no location of heavenly real estate. There is no figure that resembles a man or woman waiting for our soul to arrive. There is certainly no Pearly Gate with Saint Peter taking admission tickets. There is no humanlike figure with horns coming out of his head and a tail and a pitchfork waiting for you in a burning hell, either. These are myths.

There is no Santa Claus.

Let us begin a serious discussion meant for adults.

Many of the writings held in reverence by religions worldwide have truth in them. The meaning gets lost. Why? When it is written as clearly as the quote in the Gospel of Luke where to find the Kingdom of Heaven, why would we look for it anywhere else? The Kingdom of Heaven is where God resides. Hence, God is there as well.

All the great spiritual teachings agree on this.

Not one of the masters - Jesus, Krishna, Buddha, Mohammad, Moses, or Lao Tzu - ever suggested there is a location anywhere else but within us. Yet all religions of mankind give the wrong directions to the Path of Eternal Life. Why that is so is not our concern. Pondering a lie gets us no closer to the truth.

People point upward because that is the general location of the higher chakra everyone possesses, where is found connection to the ether and heavens and the Source, where all knowledge resides.

We agree almost universally that there is an inner self. We are more than flesh and bones. And there is a general consensus that the principle of eternity and eternal life are valid and real. The beliefs in which there is nearly universal agreement lead to the conclusion that that which is within us is eternal. We live forever after we have exhausted the physical body.

The English word for that which is eternal within us is soul. The soul we cannot locate physically. The mind is the same. We have another word. The word is psyche. And we have no physical location for where the psyche is either.

The Merriam-Webster Dictionary offers "soul" as a synonym for "psyche" and "personality" as a synonym for "mind." Given this definition, we now know that the mind, the soul, and the psyche are all the same and interchangeable in language. Yet each word conjures a different image, a different representation, a different mask, when spoken or read.

If I were to speak before a church congregation and say the Lord will save your psyche, how long would the congregation allow me to speak? Not long at all is correct.

Because the intention of this chapter is to provide information without segregation, the three words will be written as mind-soul-psyche or its acronym, MSP.

The discussion from here onward will be centered on the functions of the mind-soul-psyche. What are the components of the MSP, and how can we utilize fully the powers it gifts to us freely?

Now that we understand the mind being the soul being the psyche as one, we must come to further understanding of this phenomenon of the self that we cannot locate but agree exists.

The MSP has three workings.

A. There is the conscious state of being. When in the conscious state, we use all our senses.

We use all the senses that we have ability to use. Sight, Touch, Hearing, Smell, and Taste. The five senses are how we experience the physical world.

B. There is the unconscious state of being. In this condition, the mind and body are at complete rest. We do not intentionally use the five senses. Fortunately, hearing, touch, and smell remain functional enough to alert of disturbances that might be threatening to life or limb, like a gunshot or smoke from a fire in the kitchen. In this unconscious state of being, if we hear something, if we smell something, if we feel something, we return to the conscious being. We wake up to see what is going on. What touched us? What smells so strongly? What is that noise?

C. There is the subconscious state of being. This is where we will spend considerable discussion in this chapter. We know this level of consciousness exists because we dream. We all dream. Some people do not remember dreaming and will say, "I don't dream," but they are wrong. Others of us are very engaged with dreaming. The occurrence of dreaming is intermittent. Dreaming only occurs during certain sleep cycles. Dreaming is associated with the period in the cycle of sleep when there is Rapid Eye Movement (REM). During dreams, our senses are active. We see, we hear, we speak, we touch and feel and taste, and we experience emotion. Fear, surprise, lust, and every other emotion is available in our dreams.

That all our five senses are active and available to the subconscious in our dreams is very interesting, even fascinating.

We go to new places and to familiar places. We see people we currently know and others we have known in our life, and we also meet strangers. People we have never met show up in our dreams and we form relationships with these people. Sometimes, the relationship is adversarial and, at other times, very cordial and occasionally intimate. We see animals, trees, buildings, waterways and, oceans, and mountains. We have the sensations of flying and of falling. We even think about the situations and circumstances that are before us. We are

179

thinking in our dreams. We may ask questions like, Should I follow this person or not? Why am I attracted sexually to this person when we only met in this dream moments ago? We might even see someone familiar but whom we only know from our dreams. We will greet them with familiarity, as we would greet a friend or lover in conscious reality.

And it is our personality in our dreams. It is us. Our MSP (mind-soul-psyche) is experiencing another reality. We realize the dream state allows us to enter a separate reality. We carry our personality and memories and all our senses into dreams. We can have such vivid dreams that we believe what is happening is real. Our dreams are a life experience. This life experience is that of the subconscious. The subconscious is where we have access to our mind. The subconscious is where we have access to our soul. The subconscious is where we have access to our psyche.

And we can control this experience. We can control our mind, and so we have control of the psyche and soul. We have complete control.

We have theorized that eternal heaven is within us. Now, we have determined that we will experience another reality in our dreams. We have also found that silence in prayer and meditation is essential to reach this subconscious: our deeper consciousness. Remember, it is an inside job. That is why prayer and meditation is performed in silence.

It is through prayer and meditation that we strengthen our communication and connection with the subconscious. And this is where intuition dwells and surfaces in sudden bursts of inspiration, or as a premonition of things to come, or of unexplainable "feelings" about what to do about a situation or a person. We are attracted and repulsed by instinct, a sense of like or dislike. This is intuition coming to us from the subconscious to help us in situations of consequence in the waking physical conscious world we call reality.

Dr. Glenn Livingston of the Coach Certification Alliance offers this statement in his training materials:

Intuition is a feeling about something (or some-one) which is instinctive and sometimes beyond reason. We experience intuition as a hunch, which can appear to come completely out of the blue.

Livingston theorizes that intuition is information coming from storage in the unconscious. My theory is that intuition comes from information gathered and stored in the subconscious.

Either way, we can come to rely on our intuition as we develop access to it. Like any muscle, if we exercise it and use it, it will strengthen.

Merriam-Webster clearly has a definition that supports what has already been written here.

The formal word definitions do not make the connection with the subconscious. That is not the role of a dictionary. Merriam-Webster states that intuition is a natural ability or power that makes it possible to know something without any proof or evidence: a feeling that guides a person to act a certain way without fully understanding why.

If prayer and meditation strengthens this inborn and natural human ability, then why not develop it. Just as we would expand our knowledge of a specific subject by studying, or build muscles to lift greater weight or run faster or a greater distance.

Communication and a relationship with our subconscious through meditation will allow our intuition to bring us greater insight and more inspiration than we ever thought possible.

By definition, we will possess:

1: quick and ready insight

2a: immediate apprehension or cognition, b: knowledge or conviction gained by intuition, and c: the power or faculty of attaining to direct knowledge or cognition without evident rational thought and inference

Where does the subconscious get the information that informs the intuition, that, in turn, informs us consciously? Consider the following summation: "[The] collective unconscious is the part of the collective psyche that is unconscious, the other parts being consciousness of the perceptible world and consciousness itself." This brief statement is drawn from the research of Swiss psychiatrist Carl Jung into the psyche. In his work, Jung theorized a collective psyche.

We have already determined that "psyche" is synonymous with "mind" and "soul," and so the phrases "collective soul" and "collective mind" are acceptable terms. Being that our interest here is spiritual and not psychological, we can contemplate a collective MSP (mind-soul-psyche). Understand that neither a psychiatrist nor a psychologist can explore their research as a spiritual quest. Just as a speaker cannot claim to a church congregation that the Lord will save our psyche, neither can the psychologist write that he or she is researching the soul. Their profession must use the word psyche.

Here, we are not limited by these semantic differences and word games.

Jung puts forth in theory that there is a collective unconscious. Then reason follows there would exist a collective conscious and a collective subconscious.

A. The individual conscious communicates with the collective conscious.

B. The individual subconscious communicates with the collective subconscious.

The collective is comprised of the consciousnesses of all humankind.

And when the subconscious is dreaming it is dreaming with the collective subconscious, where we all are dreaming together. That is who these people are that we meet in our dreams. They are other personalities that exist in the past, present, or future, and they are in the now-moment of our dream state.

Just as we mingle socially with one another in conscious contact in reality on this physical earth, the subconscious mingles in the world of the ethereal. When we meet on earth a familiar and friendly person, we intuitively feel connected, and when there is a sense of romance then we believe we have met our soul mate.

Merriam-Webster defines "ethereal" as: in heaven and resembling heaven; seeming to belong to another world.

Specifically:

1a: of or relating to the regions beyond the earth-bound: celestial, unwordly, and spiritual

2a: lacking material substance: immaterial: suggesting the heavens or heaven

And the word "ether" is, by definition the sky -the heavens - the upper regions of space.

Note that the word spiritual is included in the above definition 1a. We know (in this theory) that the God we seek is within us, and we know that we possess a subconscious that brings us dreams and intuition. We know that the spiritual is celestial and so beyond.

If you have followed this line of reasoning thus far, then that is sufficient for us to go forward imaginatively into the ether, where our subconscious finds the information that informs our intuition. Therefore, intuition is defined as it is a feeling that guides without rational understanding about why.

It is apparent in our language. Any and every time we experience an inspired moment, a sudden intuitive insight, we are surprised and in awe. That is intuition. We may just say, "Wow!" or often (even an atheist may) exclaim, "Oh, my God!" Inspired moments happen. Inspire is a word from the French language; it means in spirit. When we are inspired we have connected to the universal spirit: the cosmos. We are in spirit.

Intuition and inspiration are both experiences we have that come from the subconscious.

You will be surprised when the answer springs forth intuitively. In an epiphany, the answer will stare you in the face. Why? This happened because, if only a few moments, you gave the subconscious time in silence for the truth to surface to light or fall from out of the blue. (Use whichever analogy works for you.)

Ether is what we live in. We breathe it. The wind is in the ether. The stars are in the ether. All is in the ether.

Ether is defined as 1) the upper regions of space; the clear sky; the heavens, 2) the medium supposed by the ancients to fill the upper regions of space, 3) a hypothetical substance supposed to occupy all space, postulated to account for the propagation of electromagnetic radiation through space.

Synonyms for the word ether are "air," "atmosphere," and "sky." Atmosphere has the synonym "heaven." A synonym for sky is "firmament," and for firmament is "space."

"Blowin' in the Wind," written by Bob Dylan (which became an anthem for social activism in the 1960s), contains the lyric "the answer is blowing in the wind," states directly that in the wind, which blows in the ether, are all answers. The impact of this song was socially inspiring; it moved millions. I am sure it came as intuitively inspired insightfulness to Bob. Either that or he thought long and hard about the philosophy of the Source of knowledge. Here is an excerpt.

How many roads must a man walk down

Before you call him a man?

Yes, 'n' how many seas must a white dove sail

Before she sleeps in the sand?

Yes, 'n' how many times must the cannon balls

fly

Before they're forever banned?

The answer, my friend, is blowin' in the wind

The answer is blowin' in the wind.

Silence

"A great many people think they are thinking when they are merely rearranging their prejudices."

-**William James**, 19th century philosopher

When I Was In Madrid, Spain, In 1971, It Was Very Peculiar For Me To Find That Daily Afternoon Siesta Was A Common Practice. All Shops And Business Closed For About Three Hours. After Siesta, They Return To Work Until As Late As Ten O O'clock At Night.

Businesses in Paris, France, would take a three-hour lunch, and there, too, people would work till late in the evening. In London, England, they still had afternoon teatime.

These cultural practices force everyone to slow down.

Our American culture rarely slows down. The majority of people in the United States eat fast, drive fast, and walk fast, and when we relax it is as an individual. This "down time" is spent looking at a cell phone, surfing the Internet, searching for music, watching TV programs or movies. The American mind and consciousness gets little to no quiet, no peace. Is this why alcohol drinking and drug use are so prevalent? Is this the only way Americans slow down and get silence?

Outside stimulation every waking hour is not needed to live a happy life.

When we are in silence then the Universe can connect to us without distraction. Then, we can consciously listen to what is going on in our mind with awareness. Our subconscious has no interference in connecting to the Source that exists in the ether. So, communication is made strong and clear. That's the communication that prayer and meditation allows: getting connected. These activities allow access to our intuitive self.

These practices also reinforce the experience of living in the now-moment.

The Source communicates to us in silence. That is the purpose of silence: to hear and listen to that which dwells within us. Silence is the language of the Source. The Source is God, and God is within and so we need quiet. Silent solitude is how we find what the Source has to share. We need silence in abundance. We grow in enlightenment this way.

American culture does not encourage silence or enlightenment.

Quite the opposite is true - our society promotes chaos, confusion, crisis, sexual ecstasy, fantasy, drinking and drugging, drama and noise. Most people believe they are bored unless being stimulated with a distraction. Many believe auditory (loud music) or visual (big-screen TVs) noise is necessary for happiness.

It was less than a century ago that not even a radio could be found in a home. And when we got radios into homes, there were only programs at certain times of day. Then along came television, and again there was only programming for so many hours each day. Then came color television and stereo sound, and Americans were thrilled!

Most people cannot imagine not having television, a tablet or a laptop and a smart phone today. Even vehicles have become barriers between us and silence.

Certainly, do we all not wish for peace and quiet at times? It is part of our vernacular, our lingo.

When we say, "I need some quiet and time to think," that is the voice of our MSP (mind-soul-psyche). It is surfacing to our conscious consciousness and shouting to be heard.

Silence may not be easy to get used to. Our culture has not taught us to appreciate silence. But there is no doubt that psychologically we need it. Let it be stated in a way that may make it very clear.

The Source God is a psychological necessity to the human condition. The Source is not an imaginary man in the sky. The Source is within us and beyond us, and we must be in communication, we need to know this oneness, for without this relationship, we go insane.

Unfortunately, from what I see, it is too late.

It seems that sanity, to a large extent, has clearly left our streets, schools, and systems of justice and society.

Give it a try. Be quiet. Put silence back in your life and it nourishes your soul. There is no such thing as absolute silence; we can only strive to get as close as we can to it. We need silence to understand ourselves and to develop a relationship with the Source.

This will give you a chance to work on one of the virtues you found lacking within you, which you wrote in your exit strategy journal. Growing accustomed to losing your addiction noise and outside stimulation will take time. Patience for many must be acquired because we have become so accustomed to the hustle-and-bustle way of life.

Being in silence, you grant yourself time to be at peace, serene, and reflective. Begin with gratitude and appreciation for this opportunity to begin a sober life.

Leave the electronic distractions off frequently.

Do this more and more often, and you will come to appreciate silence. You cannot listen to your inner voice and talk at the same time. Take control of your mind and your space.

What we have learned is that intuition is also known as the sixth sense.

Dreams come from our subconscious.

The subconscious never sleeps. We know the subconscious exists because we dream. And in dreams, we are having experiences. We feel fear, pleasure, and happiness. We see strangers and, animals, and loved ones in our dreams. We go to places new and to locations familiar. Through the experiences of thoughts and emotions in our dreams, we receive information. This information is stored in the subconscious.

Our subconscious can be accessed and strengthened purposefully. Through meditation, we become acquainted with our subconscious consciously. Gaining access to our subconscious brings intuitive thought. Intuition is strengthened through meditation till we come to rely on it.

Developing conscious contact with our subconscious makes the sixth sense stronger.

Sixth-sense, right-brain intuition provides premonitions and even clairvoyance. Intuition is instinctual. Intuition is what early humankind used to survive before ration or reason. Those ancient ancestors survived with intuitive instinct.

Everyone has the capacity for intuition. In this modern world, we do not seek to develop it. Why? Is it because we think our left-brain, rational intellect is superior to instinctual intuition?

Generally, we never let our inner voice get a word in edgewise. By never letting silence surround us, we miss serenity, and sanity remains elusive. We do not pause. We make snap decisions with little thought, if any. We talk over and at others and call it a conversation.

We are too busy distracting ourselves with pleasure and instant gratification with sex, drugs, money, movies, games, and smart phones. And the latest fashion is crucial to being accepted by others. Our appearance is so important - we say, "I need to take another selfie," and then immediately text or tweet, "Do you like me now?" Seeking admiration of others, we stroke our ego, pleased when we receive a compliment.

We do not love ourselves with this behavior.

Giving yourself time in silence allows you to get to know you. It may be uncomfortable at first. But with practice, you will learn how to control the thoughts of your mind. When negative thoughts occur, you will detect them and know to change them to positive. This is why the disciplines of repeating positive affirmations, prayer, meditation, and journal writing, including making gratitude lists and even to-do lists, are important. Using these tools will allow you to develop greater and ever-increasing control of your mind. You will, in the process, come to know yourself. And because you are sober, right-brain intuitive skills will increase in their dependability.

There is an adage that goes, "Who feels it knows it." Intuition is coming to know without reason.

Intuition produces premonitions. The sixth sense provides revelation through insight. A premonition is the anticipation of an event without conscious reason.

Have you ever been with someone that has the same thought at the same time? Two of you have the same intuitive premonition simultaneously? The subconscious of each of you has drawn from the ether at the same time. You look at each other, and with the look in each other's eyes, you know the other knows what you know.

The collective consciousness is where everyone's subconscious resides. The collective subconscious draws true information from the ether when the mind is clear: free of mind-altering drink or drug. You are thinking that is quite an extraordinary concept, right? Then answer me this. When good information, truthful knowledge, comes suddenly to mind, where do you think that came from?

No. You did not just think of it. You were not thinking at all. You were eating ice cream in the park, watching a squirrel fuss with an acorn, when suddenly, a notion entered your consciousness. You got the sudden thought, "He is cheating me!"

That was an intuitive thought, out of the blue ether.

The next logical and intuitive thought is, "Oh, so now I understand. That's why..." And you know it. But you don't want to believe it. So maybe you even brush it off as a silly notion, dismiss the possibility that it could be true.

Or you can convince yourself that it is true.

At that moment, on the park bench, you need to decide. Thank goodness you are in a silent place in the park, so you can breathe and calm your mind. Everything there is to know is in the ether. You are silent long enough while sitting in the park to have an intuitive thought. And now you believe you know what is going to happen in the future. Your intuition has become dependable because you are sober.

If, in the park, you had been talking and texting and taking the thirteenth "selfie" of the day, your subconscious could not have gotten through to you. Your intuition is blocked by the overload of visual and auditory noise.

Intuitive knowledge comes easier with a clear mind and less distraction.

Intuition comes through the right brain, and the left brain has to rationally decide how best to use the information.

Let's say a friend asks for a ride to a place, and you know you shouldn't bother. You are on your way to work or to pick up a child. The friend pleads with you about the urgency of their plight. You surrender your will to them. Your intuition said not to do this. But you ignore it.

After all, it's on the way. Then, after you are on the road, your friend asks, "Do you mind if we stop in here?"

"What the hell?"

"It will only take a minute." And the minute becomes ten long anxious minutes. Now you have become frustrated and stressed because you are late to attend to your own affairs. And you think, "I should have followed my gut feeling." That was a sudden premonition that you missed.

You are not being selfish when you cannot accommodate someone else's desires. You are doing no harm to you. You do come first. Got it? When your mind is clear, and your actions are sober.

As true as water is wet, silence is golden.

Write On

"One's own thought is one's world. What a person thinks is what he becomes. This is the eternal mystery."

The Upanishads (800-600 BC)

Integrate Enjoyable Activities Into Your Life.

Doing things, you love that are life affirming is how you love yourself. Self-love is essential to wellness. Think of practicing silence as an activity. Incorporate prayer, meditation, and journal writing into your daily quiet time. You can come to enjoy these activities, and getting to know the real you is the reward. And now you get to know you with a clear mind!

Prayer and meditation have been emphasized in earlier chapters. Now, let's get the write on.

Write how you really feel. No one will read your journal without your permission. Don't write for posterity, to be memorialized. Leave that ego-driven nonsense to the likes of presidents, captains of industry, and military commanders. You don't want to be, and it is unlikely you will ever be, like these men. Then again, maybe you could become a captain of industry. Anyone can be president.

Captain of industry, I like that goal.

You write this goal into your journal and in your exit strategy notebook. You begin to make plans to become a captain of the renewable-energy industry. And you remind yourself that unless your mind is clear and you are sober, you cannot achieve this goal.

You have written into your journal this goal. Now, write down how you feel right now. And you write into your journal, "I feel excited right now. I feel enthusiastic!"

You made a great journal entry. You wrote what happened. You set a goal. And you wrote how you felt at that very now-moment. You expressed those emotions on paper with the physical motion of writing, which strengthens the forces working toward the goal.

Make sure to date the entry.

Keep this journal simple and part of your day.

It only took fifteen minutes to do that entire process.

Another thing not to do is to write while thinking about your spouse, children, or grandchildren. This will cripple your freedom of expression. You are writing for self-knowledge and spiritual growth, mental and emotional health. You love yourself by being true to yourself.

The writing you are doing is a tool to help you stay sober.

Go ahead and express the frustration, grief, and depression you feel as you shed an old way's life in addiction and it is buried. Those feelings are common and normal and it is important to write this in your journal.

Expressing gratitude or elation and joy to be beginning a sober life and enthusiasm for a fresh start should also be written if that is how you feel.

Everything we do, think, and feel projects energy that is either harmful or healing. Even when you express anger on a particular day, the activity of writing honestly is a soul-clearing and positive-healing activity.

Giving consciousness voice is what happens when writing a personal journal. Communicating what is truly felt inside is vital to your emotional and mental health.

Write anything that influenced your life that one day. Indicate the day and date and go about your day.

So, make silent time every day. If you are in a busy household, get quiet time for you before the others wake up or after they have all gone to bed. If you want to love you, just do it. You can do it now that you are sober.

Write about anger, sadness, and pain. Write about excitement, happiness, enthusiasm, and joy to the world. This journal is where you vent or express gratitude privately. This will lessen the anxious stress and irritability. Journaling your thoughts and feelings will increase the chances that when someone says good morning the reply they receive will not be "Get lost."

Sometimes what you write may be so painfully revealing that the anger felt then returns now and you curse aloud in your quiet place. On the other hand, perhaps a few minutes of crying with tears rolling down your cheeks, revisiting the sorrow, will be cathartic. You might laugh aloud; you may smile about something that was funny that day. Write all these thoughts and emotions down. It is liberating and therapeutic.

This is why a quiet time and a space to let silence surround you should be part of your exit strategy. Enshroud your being with positive peace. Self-knowledge increases the awareness you have, not only of self but of your social sphere.

Journal writing can lift depression as it brings clarity of mind. Do not be surprised if your intuition gives you the "aha!" moment in the middle of writing a sentence. The free-form writing that comes with personal expression unlocks creativity. Freedom to think whatever comes is creative and imaginative and allows the subconscious to communicate with the Source to you. It is much like thinking aloud or getting lost in thought. From out of the blue, an intuitively inspired idea hits you. And you may say, "Aha! Now I understand and know what to do."

This is particularly helpful for figuring things out in our relationships, business or personal. We may discover that we have not yet learned to live and let live. We have not yet learned to walk away rather than struggle. Some things can and some things cannot be fixed. Writing will help clarify what wise action should be taken.

The need to be right is something that we need to let go of, as it only leads to greater frustration and conflict. I told a woman recently, "It was cooler today than yesterday." And she shot back, "No, it wasn't. It was much hotter today." I could tell in her voice that she had to be right. Then I considered the fact that she was in another part of the city, so she could be right. Who cares about the weather? Nothing can be done about it. No reason to argue. Always keep in mind that what is important to one person never has the same importance to another. For her it was important to be right. To keep your inner peace, let the other be right if it is that important to them.

Rather than hold something inside you, write about the misunderstandings that come up. Often this will also help you understand a different point of view. Journaling also gives a greater comprehension of our own perspective. Write about your victories to bolster self-esteem.

Write when you are happy and when you are sad. When you glance through the journal from time to time you can reflect on what gave you the blues and what worked to uplift your soul, raise your spirit. You might find your own tool to keep positive energy flowing.

Psychologist James Pennebaker insists that keeping a journal has health benefits. Regular journaling, he says, strengthens immune cells. Pennebaker believes that writing about stressful stuff helps you understand better what happened and how you feel about it, and this reduces stress and ongoing worry about the situation.

Less stress cannot help but improve the immune system. Everyone knows stress makes a person vulnerable to illness. The stomach develops ulcers, the nerves are frayed, and the brain aches.

Writing allows the use of all brainpower. The right brain is free to imagine, create, and draw intuition from the subconscious and the Source, and the left brain is activated because analysis and logic must be accessed to evaluate the rationale of what is written.

Let me share some basics about the brain as science does.

Scientists have long divided the brain into categories. I don't know how they reached these conclusions, but this is the current common theory. The left brain is analytical and provides rational logic. It is used for mathematics, language, facts, computation, and words of songs. The right brain is where creativity and intuition come from, as well as imagination, feelings, and holistic thinking, rhythm, the arts, and visualization.

The frontal lobe is the part of the brain we use every day. It is said that this area of the brain controls important cognitive skills in humans: expression of emotions, problem solving, memory, language and our ability to communicate, judgment, and sexual behavior.

Don't you find it odd that judgment and sexual behavior are assigned to the same region of the brain?

People are even divided into left-brain people and right-brain people. While right-brain people may plunge head on into keeping a journal, maybe two (a diary of daily activities and a dream journal, or both included in one notebook), left-brain people might be more reluctant to express their true feelings on paper.

Here are a few tips to help those who are reluctant to get started with writing daily, once you have established quiet time during the day and are exercising silence because it is now an enjoyable activity to shut out the noise. If you live with others, waking before the household members do guarantees greater quiet time.

An example could be to routinely set aside thirty minutes at the beginning of the day, during which you practice a short prayer, fifteen minutes of meditation, and fifteen minutes of writing. These three activities set the vibration for the day in whichever order is preferred.

Writing in the morning will help wake up your brain before being bombarded with external forces and the busy business ahead. You already made a to-do list for the day the night before, so tasks and objectives are known.

Do not concern yourself with full sentences or paragraphs or grammar. Write four or five bullet points and review, and be done in five to ten minutes. This is sufficient. A few points about how you feel now and who is affecting you will suffice.

Even left-brained people can do this.

This next method is one I have used.

On a desk calendar, jot a few notes of what happened that day. Examples could be "Put the car in shop and missed work," and "Broke up with Jane.

She put a hammer in my TV."

Include in these notes how you feel. Ask yourself as you write about the emotion you felt then or now.

This method keeps a record of things that took place or how you felt about something. It is always surprising how easy it is to forget when something took place. Sometimes I think it took place two weeks ago, but it was really four weeks.

Another method could be choosing to answer

three questions every day. For instance:

1. Am I worried or enthusiastic?

2. What am I grateful for?

3. What will make this day a success?

Answer these questions or whatever questions you choose daily.

The desk calendar and three-questions methods will allow for simplicity, and the journal is just part of the day. As things come up you make note of it daily.

Right-brained people will likely have no trouble expressing their feelings about life's ups and downs. Writing will have these people use more left-brain functions, such as analysis, logic, and facts. This will cause the right-brained person to think about what they have written and are writing rationally.

Left-brained people might not believe there is good cause to expose their feelings on paper. That is why the short bullets and desk calendar methods have been suggested. If a note-taking method is chosen to ease into keeping a journal, always include a comment about the emotion the experience brought forth. For instance, "I got my car back, but I hate the bill the garage had me pay. I feel I got ripped off." And when a positive thing happens, "I finally got the pay raise and I feel great. I am excited to get back to work now!"

Once a left-brained person gets used to the practice of writing, there will be a subtle shift as the right side of their brain is awakened, and creativity, and perhaps imagination and the expression of feelings, becomes more comfortable.

However, you choose to journal, begin journaling, and begin experiencing the benefits that come from emotional expression, clarity of mind, knowledge of you, and the examination of relationships in which you participate.

Just like meditation, journaling will be most effective if you do it daily for about twenty minutes.

Again, I suggest writing by hand so you are not distracted by squiggly lines under words spelled wrong or tempted to check on Facebook friends and email. That can wait twenty minutes.

Go For It

"A goal without a plan is just a wish."

ANTOINE DE SAINT-EXUPERY, French writer, poet, journalist, and pioneering aviator.

Whatever You Desire In Life Is Likely Attainable. There Is The Gift Of Mind-Soul-Psyche Given to you at birth. This furnishes you with considerable power for self-fulfillment. This power, though, has been distorted and dulled in drunkenness and drug abuse.

Do you want to regain and keep your sacred self? Your daily intention must be to harness your power to ensure ongoing sobriety. Maintenance of personal honesty and integrity is a priority. This is the way to self-love and self-respect. Your gift of life came free and the free Source of energy flows through life, so love and respect that energy of sacred life given.

Make peace within. Be aware of your attention, intention, and focus. Sometimes, it works better to pause and consider what is being created with a certain thought or specific action. Confrontations will appear and when the challenge is there, the future you will have depends on you accepting or rejecting the challenge. When we reject challenge, we reject growth. When we fail to grow, we fail to learn, and then we cannot teach others. Learning is a responsibility of living. Accept what is before you.

You are the creator of your life.

There was a farmer who grew excellent quality corn. Every year, he won the award for the best grown corn. One year, a newspaper reporter interviewed him and learned something interesting about how he grew it. The reporter discovered that the farmer shared his seed corn with his neighbors. "How can you afford to share your best seed corn with your neighbors when they are entering corn in competition with yours each year?" the reporter asked.

"Why, sir," said the farmer, "didn't you know? The wind picks up pollen from the ripening corn and swirls it from field to field. If my neighbors grow inferior corn, cross-pollination will steadily degrade the quality of my corn. If I am to grow good corn, I must help my neighbors grow good corn."

"So, it is with our lives... Those who want to live meaningfully and well must help enrich the lives of others, for the value of a life is measured by the lives it touches. And those who choose to be happy must help others find happiness, for the welfare of each is bound up with the welfare of all."

Anonymous

When setting a goal, be very specific. And consider how others are affected as well. It is good to have a goal that benefits others as well. Your reward will always be greater with the more people you help. Your contribution to humanity and society displays the virtue of generosity.

When you set a goal, you are setting your intention. Your intention is what will manifest. Therefore, details are critical when planning to manifest a different and new reality: your thoughts form beliefs and create emotions, and this is your consciousness at work. When the consciousness is positive, so will be your actions, and actions will manifest a positive desired outcome.

Goals are not dreams.

Goals are planned. They are planned to be implemented. Big or small goals and objectives achieved and accomplished will raise your self-esteem. This makes for happiness.

By now you have written goals and objectives into your exit strategy journal. These are to be included. Know and embrace the true you. Know what you believe. Establish personal and professional goals. Live a balanced life. Build safe friendships and discard the toxic ones. Learn to live in the awareness of now. This is the way to forgive the past and not be concerned with the future.

Accept what must be decided or done. Put good energy into the thoughts and actions, and this will likely generate excitement about the tasks ahead.

Become enthusiastic and remain motivated in pursuit of your goals. Let no one deter your efforts with negativity. Reject this toxicity. When someone calls me a derogatory name, I just shake my head in amusement at their frustration. There is no need to let another person ruin my day or resolve.

Once you have prioritized your goals in order of passion and possibility, get started. Do not let procrastination stop you from doing so. Procrastination is your arch-enemy, foe, and nemesis. A relapse will derail your motivation. A drink or drug will certainly slow momentum, and procrastination is certain to prevail with a relapse, and this will end pursuit of accomplishing your goal. Now, your goal has become a dream: a pipe dream.

Why do tomorrow what can be done today? If there is an objective that requires waiting, then find some other task that can be done today toward at-taining your goal. When you think something can be done tomorrow, tomorrow tells you that there is always another tomorrow. Tomorrow never comes.

This is procrastination.

When will you conquer procrastination? The first step has been taken. You will not take that first drink today. That is accomplishment of a goal. Happiness comes with accomplishment. And you will be happy at the end of the day just doing this.

Write down the steps necessary to complete the plan. Do not fear writing. This is your consciousness speaking to you. Revealing you to yourself is what it's all about. Knowing well who you are and your objectives is all important to your exit strategy.

For instance, if you need training before you launch your business, specifics must be written down. You want to be a lawyer or a plumber, or a better husband or wife, or maybe you want a bonus at work-it's yours to decide. Plan how to achieve the objective.

The exit strategy is like a business plan. Why do you think businesses write business plans? So, they stay on track and focused on completing the objectives required to achieve the ultimate goal. The goal may be to earn $10,000,000 in the first year. If so, specific objectives must succeed. You've heard that failing to plan is planning to fail. If you don't have a written plan, you can become paralyzed with doubt and vagueness of thought, and confused in your belief. This affects your emotions and lowers your self-esteem and, thus the positive vibrations of your consciousness.

Writer Mark Twain stated, "The best way to do something great is to start now, and the best way to start now is to make a written plan, break it into small steps, and start on the first step now."

This is more reason to begin now.

Diplomat and inventor, Benjamin Franklin invented the potbelly stove. How? He did it.

Swim fins and bi-focal eyeglasses were also his inventions. Franklin did not wait for tomorrow. Of course, Ben did not have a television or Internet to surf. So, turn off the TV and, put down your smart phone and begin achieving and living your dreams.

The second thing that is vital to destroying procrastination is to quit lying. Now that you have begun a sober life, the delusions of grandeur are (or should be) being shed. Like a snake shedding its skin, a new you is entering the world. Every time you tell yourself you're going to do something and you don't, you lied to your sacred self. The way to stop believing your propaganda is to work on your plan daily. Start to fulfill and manifest your objectives now and create a new reality.

Procrastination becomes a habit just like drinking, and drugging becomes an addiction. One of the symptoms of this habit is saying, "I'll think about it," or, "I'll get back to you."

This is verbal procrastination.

Just say, "No. I cannot do that." Treat procrastination like everything else you are learning. Be selfish with your time to accomplish your goals. Do not let other people cause you to delay doing what is on your to-do list.

The hardest thing to do in destroying the procrastination habit is waiting because you are waiting to do it perfectly or at the perfect time. This trait is called perfectionism. Perfectionism will always cause delay in pursuing action.

The great World War II General George S. Patton said, "A good plan now is far better than a perfect plan next week." Patton knew something about planning. Patton led and planned battles throughout Europe.

Do not fear making a mistake. Mistakes will happen. This is how we learn. We learn from our mistakes. But we cannot learn from a mistake until we do make one. This will teach humility. This is part of becoming being a humble human instead of a vain one. Remember, this life is what you make it. And it won't always be perfect. And that is okay. Perfection only comes with practice. Practice means doing.

Diversity of interests can bring confusion and can really wreak havoc with accomplishment. Do you want to become a comedian or a singer? Do you want to be an architect, doctor, or a hairstylist? There is an old saying: "If you chase after two rabbits, you lose them both." You get lost when you have too many options. Pick a goal, make a plan, and stick to it. Follow your exit strategy. Do not become sidetracked.

Don't exclaim, "Oh! I really want to play piano professionally," when your practical goal is to run your own business as a plumber. Get one done.

After you have a successful plumbing business, then you can play piano at night. Neither will happen if you do not stay focused on one course of action.

This is why you have listed your long and short-term goals in order of priority of passion. What are the things that are most important to you? Practice focusing your attention only on the things you have heart, motivation, time, and energy for. You'll have time to do the less important things later. Let's look at the simple chores. You need to do grocery shopping because the pantry is bare, but your favorite Court TV show, Judge Judy, is coming on, and then Maury Povich, followed by Jerry Springer.

What do you do? Go get the groceries!

This leads to the next roadblock to subduing the nemesis named procrastination: indecision.

Decisions based on need and not desire or wanting lead to actions of accomplishment of tasks that make you happy. Having food for the week ahead is far greater a need than three blocks of daytime television.

You've fallen into the habit of indecisiveness, which is procrastination's greatest ally. This is the primary reason for getting your priorities straight.

"Let me think about it" is a clear indication you have not thought this out. Again, this is why making daily to-do lists and setting a schedule is so important. Once you have made clear what needs to be done and what must be done, and set a schedule, then you proceed with clarity and purpose.

Do not seek others' approval of your plans for the day or for your life. The opinion of others will not aid you on your journey. The habit of asking, "What do you think?" will often take away your dreams. Depending on who you ask. It is best to tell very few people what your ambition is because there are many who will quickly say, "You can't do that!"

Once you know where you want to be in your life in six months, just work quietly to achieve it. Make a decision about the goal, write a plan, and go for it.

Highly effective people are decisive.

The criteria for decision-making are must, need, and then desire. Ask yourself frequently, "What is the best decision I can make based on the knowledge I have?" And have no fear of accepting your intuition in making decisions. Often, your intuition knows best.

REVIEW

Have a written exit strategy plan upon release from rehab (or a treatment center, hospital, or incarceration). Focus on a few key goals and trust in your own wisdom and intuition. Set goals for something you want to achieve. Keep a daily to-do list that supports long-term goals. Keep a journal, a gratitude list, a dream journal, or all three. Acknowledge that now is the only time you can ever live. Find your support group. Find a healthy social setting. Make time for yourself doing things you enjoy. Learn to love silence and be willing to learn. Remain humble. Examine your beliefs. Learn to do something meditative that you enjoy and can take with you for the rest of your life. Balance your life. Activity and serenity are both important. Do no harm to self or others. Evaluate your moral character. Correct flaws found.

Maintain a good appearance and healthy hygiene. Eat well. Live without fear. Be honest and fair. Learn patience and tolerance. Be a positive role model to others. Accept that failure is a part of the learning process. Accept that life is a journey.

Practice forgiveness. Changing beliefs is what happens in recovery. The attainment of righteous principles is the goal. Believing that your life is sacred is the best starting point.

Be proud of yourself. Dignity and integrity is not false pride. Be as beautiful as you are. Be confident and do what you say you will do. Being honest keeps life simple. Being true allows you to be you.

Being at one with the Source is our natural state. The gift humankind has been given is the ability to cultivate our awareness levels consciously. The point of spiritual life is to change, grow, and expand the mind. Remember what is sacred to you: family, friends, and you. Intuition can be nurtured and grow strong enough to be reliable. Do no harm. Not to others and not to you.

Remember that the goal is to gain control of your mind through sobriety and eventually be able to function successfully in society. Ignoring something is worse than forgetting. The first is intentional and maybe malicious. The latter is an innocent mistake. Do not ignore any problem.

Problems rarely go away.

Learning is happening constantly, consciously and subconsciously.

Accept that you are where you are supposed to be. Accept that because you did not plan well for your path in life, you need to correct that now. Sobriety is pain-free. Now you know what you need to do. Don't think about it. Just do it. Live sober and free, and remember that the challenges ahead are your opportunities. Taking advantage of this opportunity is your challenge.

Finding your own inner goodness is satisfying. What is good about you? Discovery is good. The goodness in one's self is why we begin a spiritual journey of seeking. This path leads to a glimpse of what we call insight or intuition. This is a significant accomplishment. We can smile as self-knowledge begins.

Bringing happiness to one's self is such a joy to have. Then we become abundant, and then giving to another becomes irresistible. We have too much love to hoard. Sharing supplies the heart with purpose in our mind-soul-psyche. We experience a light - enlightenment - self-knowledge. Self-recognition is being fulfilled. Instead of seeking what to take - seek what can be given.

Love yourself and go for all life offers!

Appendix

References and Recommended Reading

Balch, Phyllis A., C.N.C. Prescription for Nutritional Healing: A Practical A-to-Z Reference to Drug-Free Remedies Using Vitamins, Minerals, Herbs & Food Supplements. New York: Avery, 2010.

Berger, Allen, Ph.D. 12 Hidden Rewards of Making Amends. Center City, MN: Hazelden Publishing, 2013.

Campbell, T. Colin, Ph.D., and Howard Jacobson, Ph.D. Whole: Rethinking the Science of Nutrition. Dallas, TX: BenBella Books, 2014.

Campbell, T. Colin, Ph.D., and Thomas M. Campbell II, M.D. The China Study: The Most Comprehensive Study of Nutrition Ever Conducted and the Startling Implications for Diet, Weight Loss, and Long-Term Health. Dallas, TX: BenBella Books, 2006.

Carlson, Richard, Ph.D. Don't Sweat the Small Stuff...And it's All Small Stuff. New York: Hyperion, 1997.

Celebrate Recovery. http://www.celebraterecovery.com

Chopra, Deepak. God: A Story of Revelation. New York: HarperOne, 2013.

Chopra, Deepak. The Third Jesus: The Christ We Cannot Ignore. New York: Harmony, 2009.

Covey, Stephen R. The 7 Habits of Highly Effective People: Powerful Lessons in Personal Change. New York: Free Press, 2004.

Dowrick, Stephanie. Seeking the Sacred:

Transforming Our View of Ourselves and One Another. New York: TarcherPerigee, 2011.

Ed. James H. Hutson. The Founders on Religion: A Book of Quotations. Princeton, NJ: Princeton University Press,

2007.

Epstein, Greg M. Good Without God: What a Billion Nonreligious People Do Believe. New York: William Morrow, 2010.

Feiling, Tom. Cocaine Nation: How the White Trade Took Over the World. Cambridge, UK: Pegasus, 2012.

Fernandez, Humberto, and Therissa A. Libby, Ph.D.

Heroin: Its History, Pharmacology, and Treatment.

Center City, MN: Hazelden Publishing, 2011.

Foods That Harm, Foods That Heal. New York: Readers Digest, 2004.

Frawley, Dr. David. Ayurveda and the Mind: The Healing of Consciousness. Delhi, India: Motilal Banarsidass, 2005.

Gorski, Terence T. Understanding the Twelve Steps: An Interpretation and Guide for Recovering. Fireside, 1991.

Hamer, Dean H. The God Gene: How Faith is Hardwired Into Our Genes. New York: Anchor, 2005.

Hill, Napoleon. Think and Grow Rich. CreateSpace Independent Publishing Platform, 2014.

"J." A Simple Program: A Contemporary Translation of the Book Alcoholics Anonymous. New York: Hyperion, 1996.

Kethcham, Katherine, and William F. Asbury. Beyond the Influence: Understanding and Defeating Alcoholism. New York: Bantam, 2000.

Kilham, Chris. Psyche Delicacies: Coffee, Chocolate, Chiles, Kava, and Cannabis, and Why They're Good for You. Emmaus, PA: Rodale, 2001.

King, Deborah. Be Your Own Shaman: Heal Yourself and Others With 21st-Century Energy Medicine. Carlsbad, CA: Hay House, 2012.

Lee, Martin A. Smoke Signals: A Social History of Marijuana. New York: New York: Scribner, 2013.

McCraw, Dr. Margaret. The Relationship Code: Engage and Empower People With Purpose and Passion. Wayne, NJ: Career Press, 2010.

McGowan, Kat. "Meet the Super Taskers." Psychology Today. Jan. 1, 2014.

Okrent, Daniel. Last Call: The Rise and Fall of Prohibition. New York: Scribner, 2011.

Osteen, Joel. Your Best Life Now: 7 Steps to Living at Your Full Potential. New York: Hachette: 2004.

Pluymen, Bert. The Thinking Person's Guide to Sobriety. New York: St. Martin's Griffin, 2000.

Reding, Nick. Methland: The Death and Life of an American Small Town. New York: Bloomsbury USA, 2010.

Religion Facts. http://www.religionfacts.com

Renard, John, Ph.D. The Handy Religion Answer Book. Beauty in Canton Township, MI: Visible Ink Press, 2001.

Rosen, Rebecca, and Samantha Rose. Spirited: Unlock Your Psychic Self and Change Your Life. New York: HarperCollins, 2011.

Ryan, M. J. The Power of Patience: How to Slow the Rush and Enjoy More Happiness, Success, and Peace of Mind Every Day. New York: Harmony, 2003.

Shaynebance. "History of Yoga: A Complete Overview of the Yoga History." Awaken. Dec. 15, 2015.

Simmons, Russell. "3 Simples Ways Meditation Will Make You a Better Entrepreneur."

Entrepreneur. March 18, 2014.

Spiritual Research Foundation.

http://www.spiritualresearchfoundation.org.

The New Oxford Annotated Bible With Apocrypha: New Revised Standard Version. Oxford, UK: Oxford University Press, 2010.

Tolle, Eckhart. A New Earth: Awakening to Your Life's Purpose. New York: Penguin, 2008.

Trimpey, Jack. Rational Recovery: The New Cure for Substance Addiction. New York: Gallery Books, 1996.

Tutu, Desmond, and Mpho Tutu. The Book of Forgiving: The Fourfold Path for Healing Ourselves and Our World. New York: HarperOne, 2014.

Zukav, Gary. The Seat of the Soul. New York: Simon & Schuster, 2014.

References and Recommended Reading: AA-Approved Books

Anonymous. Alcoholics Anonymous: The Big Book.

Alcoholics Anonymous World Services, Inc., 2002.

Anonymous. Living Sober. Alcoholics Anonymous World Services, Inc., 1980.

W., Bill. As Bill Sees It: The A.A. Way of Life. Alcoholics Anonymous World Services, Inc., 1997.

W., Bill. Twelve Steps and Twelve Traditions. Alcoholics Anonymous World Services, Inc., 2002.

About the Author

Founder of True Life Transformations, Dael is a Recovery Life Guide to people leaving rehab and struggling with alcoholism and addiction. Clients examine their personal and professional ambitions and goals in private sessions and go forward to fulfill their heart's desires in areas of their life beyond sobriety. It is Dael's experience that many persons return to their drug of choice after rehab. This occurs because there is a lack of planning for life after rehab to live a sober life. Awareness Recovery emphasizes developing an exit strategy while in rehab, or before or soon after rehab or incarceration. The emphasis is to have a plan which includes short and long term life goals. Dael believes that everyone can be happy and successful in life. He likes to say, "As true as water is wet, accomplishment and attaining goals brings happiness."